19.95

D1535662

Think
yourself
TRIM

Think
yourself
TRIM

Gloria Thomas

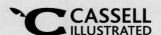

CASSELL
ILLUSTRATED

First published in Great Britain in 2003 by
Cassell Illustrated, a division of
Octopus Publishing Group Limited
2-4 Heron Quays, London E14 4JP

A CIP catalogue record for this book is available
from the British Library.

ISBN 1 84403 012 1

Design and illustrations by Tanya Devonshire-Jones
Photography by Bill Norton

Printed in Italy

Disclaimer – *It is advisable to consult a physician
in all matters relating to health and in particular to
check with your doctor before embarking on any
exercise regime. While the advice and information
in this book is believed to be accurate and true at
the time of going to press, neither the authors nor
the publisher can accept any legal responsibility or
liability for any injury sustained whilst following
the exercises.*

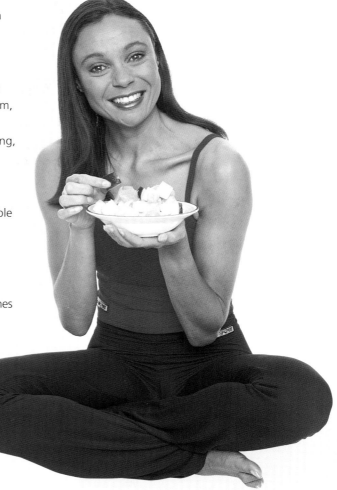

Contents

Introduction

My mother brought me up on a combination of wholesome West Indian and Irish food. It was therefore a shock when I left home to be a model and had to feed myself at the age of 18. I survived on pizzas, chips and cigarettes and all the free food that I could lay my hands on when I did promotional events. Although my diet became a little better over the years, when I became pregnant I took full advantage of the 'eating for two' myth. Towards the final stages of my pregnancy, due to complications, I found myself in hospital and literally eating for England. The result was that I put on three stones. After giving birth I suffered from a severe bout of post-natal depression and I was put on anti-depressants. I was told that I would likely be on them for life. Determined to prove the doctor wrong, I began to explore alternative ways of combating the depression and one of the ways was through food. Amazingly, all the foods that I had been eating seemed to be instrumental in the low state I was in.

I was aware that I had to make drastic changes to my diet so I decided to educate myself. Another way of dealing with the way I was feeling was through physical fitness so I then trained and became a fitness instructor. Not only did I get fit, which got rid of any excess weight, but my new found energy also taught me how to motivate others and help them to reach their goal weight. I became aware of how clients used food as a method of coping with life's stresses and strains. From fitness I moved into personal and human development to get a greater understanding of myself and the world around me. I explored new disciplines such as NLP, hypnotherapy and healing. My life's experiences have brought about a transformation within me and I now offer you the tools I developed from my experience so you can do the same. This book invites you to explore your experience with diet culture and offers insight into how food, emotions and behaviour are linked and how you can make changes to transform your own experience. Bon appetit!

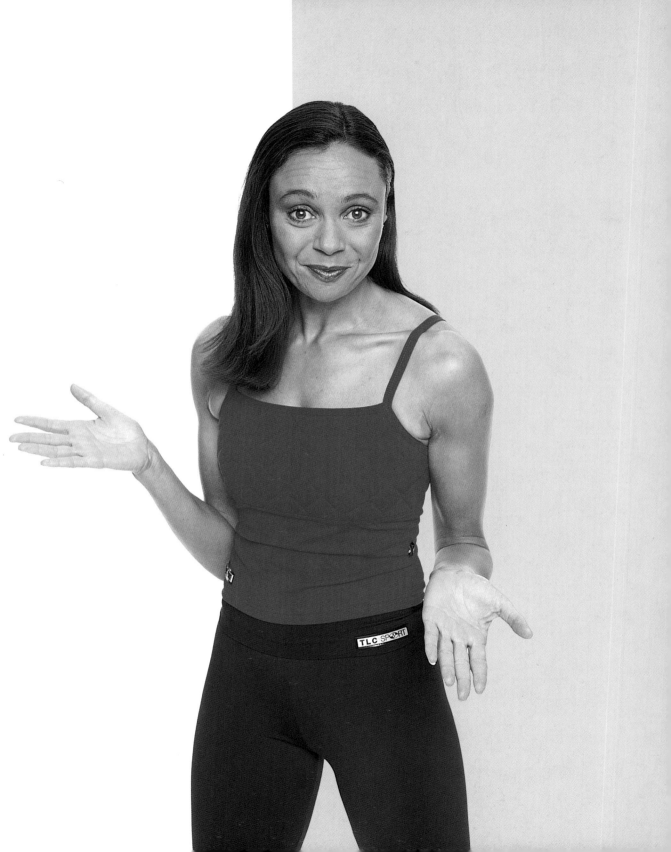

Chapter 1

Food and Eating Today

Why is it that we are so obsessed with our bodies? How is it that some people can manage their weight easily and without effort and others can't? Why does some people's weight seem to go up and down like a yo-yo? What are compulsive and binge eating? Why do our emotions seem to affect our bodyweight? How are mood and food related? What effect has diet culture had on our eating patterns? And will there ever be a magical formula for losing weight?

Food and Eating Today

The answers to these questions – and many more – can be found in this book. Your experience of eating, the way you react to food, your attitude to life, the way you handle your emotions, and the way you have been programmed to think are all likely to affect your eating patterns. Believe it or not you weren't born with your current eating behaviour. You didn't come into this world chomping on chocolate bars or tucking into large portions of chips with a generous slice of cheesecake for pudding. Over time you have cultivated and learned the eating behaviour that you have today. That process of learning most likely started within your social environment: you have been heavily influenced by family and friends and you have already been hypnotized by the society that you live in. You are today the product of your experiences yesterday – whether those experiences were positive or negative. The result of those experiences you wear on your body. 'You are what you eat' is true in every sense.

You Are What You Eat

For some people this is a happy thought – they have a good relationship with food and manage and handle their eating well. But for others there is a darker side. It may be that your eating patterns are spiralling out of control; you may eat compulsively; your way to resolve difficulties may be to stuff emotions down by shoving a cream cake in your mouth; you may have simply adopted poor eating habits over the years; you may have an unconscious need for insulation in the form of excess weight to protect yourself from life; you may have some form of disordered eating pattern. If this is the case then don't worry: the great news is you can change your existing relationship with food if you choose to. You can explore your experience for a greater awareness and insight into your existing eating patterns. You can learn and develop a new attitude towards eating. Food need not hold you to ransom or have a vice-like grip on your emotions. In the same way that you have learned your current food behaviour you can unlearn it and re-educate yourself for a new approach to eating.

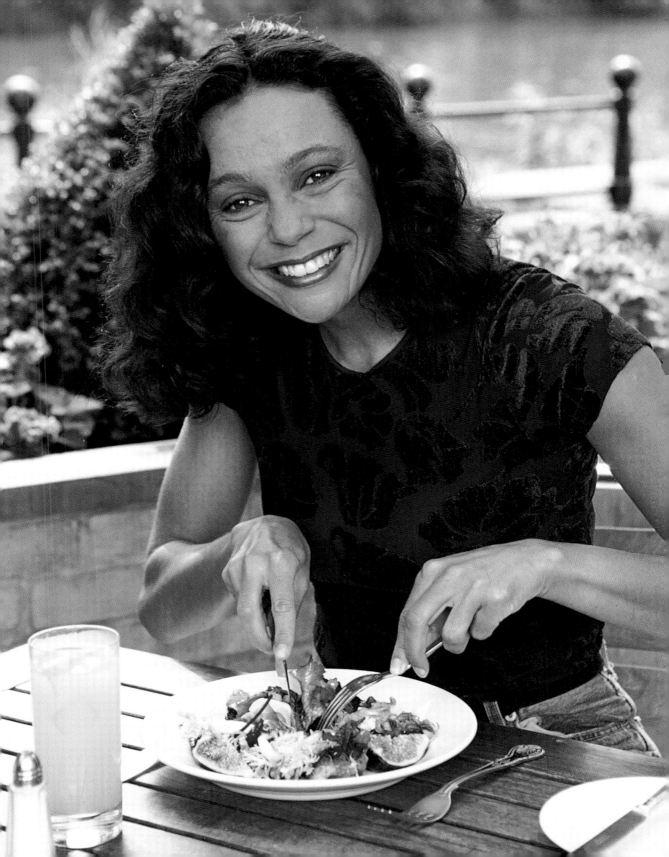

A Different Approach

The way you think, your perception and interpretation of events can lead to success or failure in life. In the past you might have allowed your conditioned mind to control you but now you can take control and train your brain. Disciplines such as neuro-linguistic programming, accelerated learning and hypnotherapy have given us the potential to do this. These disciplines and many more have given us the framework to enable us to explore our experiences and improve our understanding of how the mind works and how we process information; and, most important, they open up ways to make deep, lasting changes quickly and easily. Perhaps the most important thing to realize is that we have the most incredible resources within us to achieve our dreams in life. We just need to learn how to tap into them. And first it is essential to explore your food experience to date.

We live in a society in which food is available in abundance. Processed food is loaded with excess sugar and salt to tempt the taste buds and make us buy more. Genetically engineered food, organic food, fresh food and food from all over the world is there for us to feast on. Food is designed and marketed in line with current trends and fashions, and wrapped up in enticing packages. Healthy eating – food for the heart and for cholesterol levels – are promoted everywhere. Where weight management is concerned, there are low-fat alternatives to help you slim, and foods low in calories so you can have more of them!

Delicious foods are advertised everywhere, on billboards, in magazines, on the television and radio. We have been conditioned in the same way that Russian physiologist Pavlov conditioned his dogs. A ringing bell was a signal that food was on its way and the dogs salivated in expectation! It is the same for us. As human beings, we respond to images we see and hear – images that flood our minds with the memories of the taste and smell of immaculately prepared dishes. We hear catchy jingles: we all know what 'makes you work, rest and play'; which soft drink is 'the real thing'; and

In the past you might have allowed your conditioned mind to control you but now you can take control and train your brain.

who 'makes exceedingly good cakes'. We respond in the same way as animals. The anticipated taste of food triggers the flow of the digestive juices. So the next time you are in the supermarket or pass the newsagents, the remembered tastes and smells and the sight and sound of food is too much to resist – you don't stand a chance. The food is in your shopping basket and then in your mouth before you know it. Repeat this pattern a few times and before long a habit is born.

There is food in abundance around us in the West but an imbalance in the world. We have more than enough and yet a large part of the world's population is undernourished. One result of that imbalance is a Western society that is fast becoming out of control where eating is concerned. Ask yourself when was the last time you felt really hungry? You probably cannot remember. Why? Because you don't have to feel hungry anymore – food is there for the taking. This was not the case for our forefathers whose hunger motivated them to hunt for food. They never knew with certainty where the next meal was coming from. In the distant past body fat was a useful resource, used to insulate the body and for energy when food stores ran out. It is unlikely that you would have found anyone who was overweight or obese in those times. More mature readers may remember the rationing of the war years when if you didn't have a chocolate coupon you couldn't have chocolate and that was that. The result of rationing was a fitter and healthier nation.

Today in Western society you can snack to fill a gap, just to gratify yourself for a moment or two until mealtime. You have also learned to eat for reasons other than hunger. Pleasure or pain governs human behaviour. A small growl of hunger, a stressful day, an emotional blip can trigger the need to feel better through eating. Because food is so readily available our natural patterns of eating have changed: we often eat for reasons that are psychological. Our bodies are the physiological expression of our thoughts and our behaviours; and the result of the abundance of food that is available. As a result it is easy to over-consume and take in more energy than the body needs. The consequence is excess fat.

According to a recent House of Commons report, most adults are overweight and around one in five people are obese.

Environment and Culture

People's lifestyles are largely dictated by the environment and culture they live in. Western society is such that we are not required to be active anymore. We are far less active than our forefathers because today we have all the mod cons that make our lives easier and quicker. We do not use our bodies as they are naturally meant to be used.

According to a report carried out by the national audit office for the House of Commons, 'Tackling Obesity in England', most adults are overweight and around one in five people are obese – a total of eight million people in this country. The report states that in 1989, around eight per cent of women and six per cent of men were obese. Ten years on, this number had almost trebled to 21 per cent of women and 17 per cent of men. It is estimated that by 2005 a quarter of women and over one-fifth of men in England will be obese. By 2010 a quarter of all adults will be obese. According to The Obesity Awareness and Solutions Trust (TOAST) this means that every day in this country approximately 1000 people are becoming obese. How do these statistics compare with other countries in Europe?

Figures from the European Commission suggest that about 26 per cent of men and 21 per cent of women are overweight or severely overweight. Greece has the highest percentages with 35 per cent of men and 31 per cent of women in the overweight categories; in Spain it is 32 per cent of men and in Luxembourg 31 per cent, but only 17 per cent in Holland. In Portugal 31 per cent of women have a weight problem, in France 15 per cent and in Denmark 16 per cent. It has been suggested that if we continue in this way the obesity figures in this country will soon approach those in the USA. An American 'National Health' survey in 1997 showed that more than 50 per cent of US adults were overweight and, as in England, one in five were obese. Looking forward to 2030, if this trend continues the worst-case scenario is that most Americans will be obese, as will 37 per cent of the British population.

Obesity has worrying implications for health. The four most common conditions that result from obesity are heart disease, high blood pressure, diabetes (type 2) and osteoarthritis. Obesity not only seriously endangers your health, it also costs the country a lot of money. Every year around half a billion pounds is spent in patient care and a further two billion pounds is lost across the economy as a whole. It has been estimated that 18 million sick days and around 30 thousand deaths per year in this country can be linked to obesity. Deaths linked to obesity shorten life by nine years on average.

Most worrying is the thought that we may be breeding future generations of obese people. Our parents are our first hypnotists. The patterns of behaviour, perceptions and beliefs and values that we adopt in life we pass on to our children. Children's minds are like sponges in the early years of life and lifestyle habits and behaviours are formed in childhood through the messages that our parents give us. It has been recorded that children who have at least one obese parent are at higher risk of obesity. The number of obese children is growing in line with a decrease in activity and increased food consumption. Research by the British Heart Foundation reveals that in England only 55 per cent of boys and 39 per cent of girls aged 2 to 15 are active for the recommended one hour a day at a moderate intensity. It may be a cliché to say that children today are couch potatoes, sitting in front of the computer or television and living on convenience food, but it is also dangerously true.

So we are enticed and encouraged to buy and eat, and the result is that we may become overweight and in some cases obese. But you would be forgiven for thinking that in this type of society the fatter you are the happier you will be, as we are clearly being encouraged to gorge ourselves to death. However, this is in direct conflict with our society's preoccupation with appearance. In our society it is 'important' to be thin. Being fat is a social disease, and overweight individuals experience discrimination. Overweight children and adults are the subject of 'jokes' and if you are more than a little overweight our society would have you believe that you are just not attractive.

Self-image and Instinct

All cultures hold their idea of 'the body beautiful' in great esteem. (And here, for well-founded reasons, I am only going to consider the female body.) The products of thousands of years of conditioning, men – for the most part – want to procreate with beautiful, young, healthy women. Indeed, they are naturally predisposed to do so for the sake of the species and the gene pool. (This may be a generous and only partial explanation but it is fundamentally correct.) This survival-of-the-fittest-attitude is not, it hardly needs saying, the sole preserve of human beings, although the roles in the animal kingdom are often reversed. The peacock's beautiful plumage attracts the small, brown, undistinguished peahen. Stags use their magnificent antlers to fight for the favours of the females.

So we cannot blame men alone for the idealization of the female body, and neither should we. Women have equally high expectations of themselves. For women, the body is the clearest expression of self (although we don't have time or space here to consider the part conditioning plays in this). So our society – albeit often harsh and unfair – has established its ideal and exhorts individuals (implicitly and explicitly) to emulate it. Often unrealistically.

Self-image and Culture

These instincts run deep and unite humanity, although naturally different cultures have their own templates. The Romans, for example, equated fatness with wealth – if you were skinny it was not because you counted calories, but quite possibly because you were poor. So in Roman times a fuller figure was desirable. (And it is worth noting another prejudice here. In the West today weight problems are more likely to be attributed to a lack of money, to a poor diet that is financially expedient.) We all know what is meant when a woman's figure is described as 'Rubensesque', and it is clear that the voluptuous women Rubens painted reflect the tastes of his period. In Georgian England the ample bosom was in fashion. The Victorian age demanded tiny waists (women would go to incredible lengths to achieve them, even as far, it has been suggested, as having ribs removed).

However, there are other models. Some African and Arabic cultures and a number of the Polynesian islands have always preferred larger women. Today in African countries products such as 'Wate [sic] On' can be bought. Can you imagine some of the West's supermodels in one of these countries – they would be laughed at!

In the West being thin is seen as better. But West is not necessarily best. As you read the next chapter you may realise that now may be the time to question this ideal that society has pressed upon us. Perhaps we should be considering a new template for individuals to achieve: a healthy trim body shape that is acheivable for all.

We should be considering a
new template for individuals:
a healthy, trim body shape
that is acheivable for all.

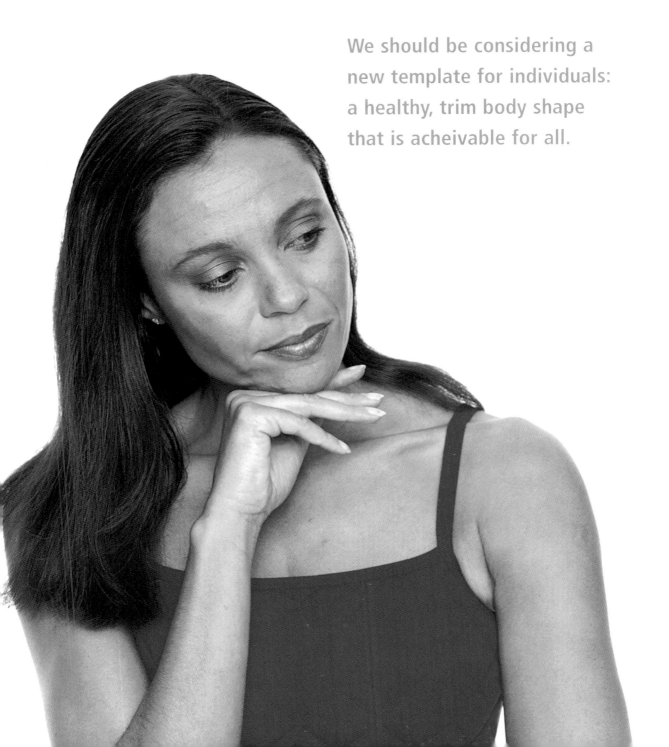

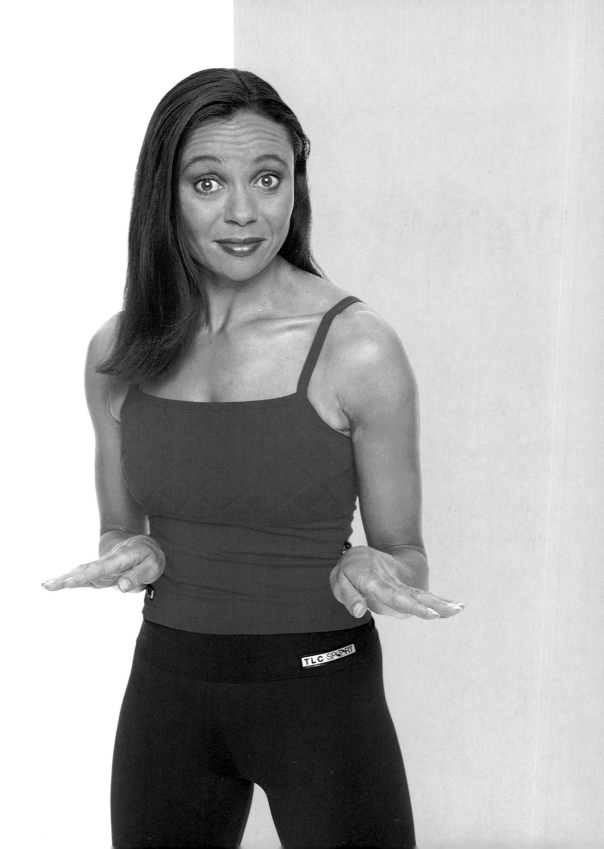

Chapter 2

Weight Control

It is clear that body shape and desirability have always been linked. But it was in the twentieth century that weight control truly became an obsession. Fundamental to this was the invention of the camera. Initially the objective of photography was primarily to register a likeness, but it became evident – especially as the reproduction of photographs became easier and more widespread – that it was going to, deliberately or otherwise, reinforce society's tastes at the same time. Photography recorded a society's ideal form and propagated it. Today the media inundates us with images of beautiful people, their flaws – such as they are – retouched by modern technology.

Weight Control

Men too began to feel the pressure. A portly body had implied wealth and social position. However, in the latter part of the nineteenth century bodybuilding – developed by a Frenchman, Edmond Desbonnet – established a new, more muscular male ideal. Photographs of the athletes and gymnasts with whom he worked were displayed in his salon, and the now traditional before-and-after pictures became familiar. Excess weight now became as desirable on men as it was on women. It was also in the Victorian age that a physician called Baird introduced the concept of dieting, and men and women became fully conscious of – even consciously focused on – the fluctuations in their weight.

Still, the curvy, hour-glass shape was all the rage until the 1950s. It is personified by the most famous of all hour-glass women: the size-14 Marilyn Monroe, then the most glamorous women in the world and even today has a powerful hold on the imagination. Trends changed in the sixties with the emergence of the supermodel (even if the name is a later coinage). The fashion industry preferred, understandably, models who showed their clothes off to the best effect and thus Twiggy the superstar was born – and so was the dieting industry, as women strove to fit into size-8 clothes. The nascent diet culture brought with it its darker side. It created anxieties, obsessions and neuroses in women who could not, they soon realized, realistically aspire to the images with which they were bombarded. They held out little hope for the average size-12 British woman. In terms of self-image – how individuals felt (or rather, were made to feel) about their bodies particularly – a corner had been turned.

In the late seventies the exercise culture was born. Not only did we have to count the calories, we also had to pound our bodies into the ground in the quest for physical perfection. Jane Fonda's revolutionary regime paved the way for other body-shape gurus. In Britain, Diana Moran and Lizzie Webb were on television every day putting us through our paces. Rosemary Conley introduced her low-fat philosophy to the world – and took it by storm. Cher, with her video *A New Attitude to Fitness*, proved that women of all ages could shape up. This process reached its culmination in the fitness videos from supermodels such as Elle McPherson and Cindy Crawford – not much to live up to there!

Unsurprisingly, the dieting and exercise industries have now developed into vast commercial businesses, making fortunes – big and very big – out of our obsession with our bodies. (Here are some figures to give you some idea of the extent of that obsession: *Time* magazine reported that 80 per cent of American children have been on a diet by the time they have reached fourth grade and that 81 per cent of Americans are afraid of becoming overweight.) All over the Western world people swear by different diets, slimming programmes and apparatus, health clubs and low-fat, low-calorie foods. If you don't, you know somebody who does.

We have seen incredible changes in our relationship with our bodies in the last hundred years or so. But – as the 'skinny period' threatens occasionally to reach its climax – it is only now sinking in that some of the extreme measures we put ourselves through to conform to the ideal work only in the short term; and that, in the long term, they carry with them a host of dangers.

Eating disorders are becoming more and more prevalent. It is estimated that 70 million people worldwide have eating disorders. They are potentially life-threatening conditions that affect men, women and children, although studies suggest that 90 per cent of sufferers are women between the ages of 12 and 25. Perhaps what we think of as the 'classic' eating disorder is anorexia nervosa, which distorts the sufferer's self-image and creates in them an aversion to food. But others are all-too-familiar:

bulimia nervosa, which sees its sufferers overeat and then vomit; and binge-eating, the sufferers of which find the urge to eat uncontrollable. (Binge-eaters are, for the record, more prone to obesity.) Again, it is interesting to note that eating disorders are almost unheard of in other societies.

Diet Culture

On the one hand, a thriving media is responsible for establishing an unrealistic ideal, and, in turn, for causing real anguish to many people who feel pressured to live up to it. On the other hand, we have an equally successful industry that exists to help you in your attempts to make and keep yourself slim, to convince you that perfection is possible. Let's take a look at what is current in the slimming market.

Calorie Restriction

It has been commonly supposed that one way to ensure weight loss is through extreme calorie restriction; in other words, greatly reducing the amount of energy that you take in. Often a crash-diet may seem, initially at least, a great success, but in truth it is not fat you are losing from your body but water and glycogen, a substance deposited in muscle tissues as a store of carbohydrates. If you continue to restrict your energy intake it will result in the breakdown of your muscle tissue for fuel – in other words, the body feeds on itself for energy!

Drastic calorie reduction can also wreak havoc with your metabolism. There are a number of physiological 'mechanisms' that we have inherited from our ancestors. One such is the famine response. When we drastically reduce what we eat the body goes into starvation mode and tells itself to start conserving fat. Your metabolism slows down in order to preserve energy and as it slows, the amount of food it requires is less. In the first

Diets don't work in the long term.

Drastic calorie reduction can wreak havoc with your metablolism.

place, to keep losing weight you need to keep eating less and less. And, secondly, when you come off your diet and resume normal eating the body, now adjusted to your lower food/energy intake, carries on in its adjusted state. Your metabolism remains slower, and your muscle mass will have decreased, and any excess calories – that is to say, what the body now perceives to be excess calories – are stored as fat. (Moreover, if you are on a restricted diet and choose to exercise you may find yourself feeling tired, weak and unable to move properly, simply because your brain and your muscles are not getting sufficient energy.)

Pills and Potions

There are many ways of restricting your calorie intake. You can, as above, cut right back on the amount of food you eat, or you can eat foods that are particularly low in calories. And you can also buy one of the many replacement meals or powdered shakes or protein drinks on the market. Again you may well lose weight quickly, but again it will be fluid and lean muscle tissue rather than fat. And the longer-term dangers are the same as well: these kinds of diets can also affect your metabolism so that when you resume normal eating you pile the pounds back on.

The medical profession has also had a role to play in the weight-loss industry. Although mainly for the clinically obese, you can get prescription pills from the doctor to suppress your appetite. One of the more popular pills are Xenical, which work by blocking the absorption of about 30 per cent of the fat that you eat. The unabsorbed fat is then eliminated in your bowel movements. But this drug can have a number of unpleasant side effects, leading to a deficiency in the fat-soluble beta-carotene (a precursor of vitamin A) and vitamins E and D. You may also suffer from flatulence and struggle to control your bowel movements – it isn't unknown (not a very nice thought this) for people not to make the toilet on time. And you need to be on a diet to use it in the first place, which begs the obvious question: which is working, the drug or the diet?

Diets can impair your metabolism.

Low-Fat Diets

Throughout the eighties and nineties the message was that we should eat well but cut out fatty foods. For some diet gurus fats were to be avoided like the plague. Less harsh programmes demanded an extreme restriction of calorie intake, low-fat diets were successful in bringing about weight loss for many people. However, nutritional science now suggests that they result in us not getting enough of the essential fatty acids – omega 3 and omega 6 – needed for body and mind to function efficiently. The right kind of fat is good for both physical and mental health. Too little fat in the diet can contribute to depressive states of mind. It has also been suggested that low fat-diets leave you feeling hungry and with cravings so that you ultimately consume more. And two low-fat chocolate puddings instead of one somehow defeats the object.

Different Types of Diet

A number of interesting eating plans have hit the market and met with a greater or lesser degree of success. 'Food combining' (originally the Hay Diet) is based on the simple rules of not mixing carbohydrates with protein and eating fruit only on an empty stomach. This has been useful for those who suffer from digestive disturbances as well as in weight loss; in fact, some people think of this as a way of eating to be adopted for life. However, most nutritionists believe that combining carbohydrates and protein isn't a cause of weight gain in the first place. Other popular diets have concentrated on restricting carbohyrdrate-heavy foods. Dr Robert Atkins' eponymous *Atkins Diet* is seen as the most aggressive of these; and while apparently successful in the short term, it has been criticized over its long-term effects. Lesley Kenton's *X-factor Diet* is a modification of the carbohydrate-focused approach, and she takes account of the fast-increasing insulin dependency that is growing in the western world. Perhaps the most interesting of eating programmes for optimum health is Dr Peter D'Adamo's *Blood Type Diet*. He believes that we all have different metabolic needs – one man's meat being another man's poison – and that people of certain blood types will thrive and feel better on certain foods, so you have to eat the foods that suit your blood group. Another variation of this philosophy is metabolic typing which suggests people have different metabolisms and therefore have different nutritional needs. I am a great advocate of these two principles. There are also many guides to nutritionally sound eating, such as *The Complete Guide to Sports Nutrition* by Anita Bean, for sportsmen and women and those who take their exercise seriously.

Extreme Measures

Most of the following are fat-reduction solutions designed for the clinically obese but they have filtered down to the 'merely' overweight and, of course, the body-conscious. Liposuction – all the rage in the nineties – involves fat being pumped out of your body, reducing excess around a given area. A tummy tuck sees fat surgically removed from your body. And if you are double your ideal (in strictly medical terms) weight, you could have your stomach stapled. In this horrific procedure four rows of staples are used to divide the stomach into a small and a large pouch, altering the way food is digested and absorbed. You could also have your jaw wired so that you can only take in fluids. And there are gastric lapbands, which require keyhole surgery, and fat magnets made out of shellfish fibres!

You could try to lose weight by going to a sauna or steam bath or by wrapping your body in fabrics that keep the heat in and make you sweat more. But, as with many of the 'cures', what you are losing is water rather than fat, and, if done too often, this can dehydrate the body. How many other methods can you think of to lose weight? Add them to this list!

The Scales

If you've tried to lose weight in the past then you've probably stepped on to the scales to measure your progress, jumping for joy if you've lost a few pounds or feeling depressed if they tell you that you've actually put on weight. However, you need to realize that you're not measuring the fat on your body (unless you have scales that are specifically designed to do so), but rather – and simply – your total body weight. You are weighing your bones, muscles, body fluids and fat – scales are not a reliable way of measuring fat. When you go on a diet you lose most weight at the beginning of that diet, but, as we've seen, this is normally fluid and lean muscle tissue. Fortunately, there are more reliable ways to measure specifically how much fat you have lost.

The Body Mass Index (BMI) is a simple and common method used to measure body fat. You calculate your BMI dividing your weight in kilograms by your height in metres squared. If you are carrying a healthy amount of fat your BMI should be between 19 and 25. If it is between 25 and 29 it means you are overweight, and anything over that is obese. So, for example, you're 1.7 metres tall and weigh 57 kilograms:

$$57/(1.7 \times 1.7)$$
$$57/2.89 = 19.75$$

... a nice, healthy BMI.

Exercise Culture

Despite the range of methods considered – the countless diets and cosmetic/surgical procedures – perhaps the best way to lose weight is still the simplest: exercise. As I mentioned earlier, exercise systems had been established long before the exercise explosion of the seventies. Indeed the Bagot Stack Exercise System, well established by the late 1920s to early 1930s, was very popular for a considerable time. Mary (but usually 'Mollie') Bagot Stack encouraged everyone to overcome conflicts by setting 'flesh against spirit or spirit against flesh' to encourage people to overcome conflicts about exercise – a true mind-body approach that was way ahead of its time. 'Little do we realize the delight that awaits us when we have trained our body to be our own instrument on which we play our part in the great orchestra of life.' Today, just over 70 years later, there are health clubs and gyms everywhere offering such an incredible range of activities that everyone can find a way to enjoy being active and actively managing their weight. There's sophisticated cardio equipment and the now familiar aerobics and step classes. You can salsa and line-dance yourself trimmer. There are spinning studios and aquaclasses in the pool – a constant stream of new ideas and techniques.

You occasionally hear the argument that gyms are not natural. Well, it is far better to be 'unnatural' than unfit. We should be using our bodies (they are designed for activity) but most of the time our society does all it can to encourage us not to. TOAST has said that 'Obesity was thought of as an abnormal response to a normal environment; obesity is becoming a normal response to an abnormal environment.' In other words, when our environment demanded that we were fit and active (making fitness 'normal'), obesity stood out as anomalous; today, with our 'abnormal' environment encouraging inactivity and excessive consumption of food, obesity and weight problems are becoming the new norm. And, as we've seen from the figures given earlier, if we continue this way and if the environment doesn't change or we don't – obesity will escalate further.

However, if you have any sympathy with the idea that gyms are unnatural, or you are at all put off or intimidated by them, be reassured that there is so much you can do without going near a health club. Try walking, running, swimming, dancing, cycling, and home-exercise videos (*see* the exercises in chapter 6, p. 124).

Energy In

So, on the one hand eating too much means – obviously – that we put on weight, but on the other hand not eating enough leads to weight gain in the long term as the body's starvation response kicks in. What to do? The answer, I believe, is to address both the quality and the quantity of energy that we take in. Clearly you need to restrict your calorie intake to a certain degree to achieve weight loss, but you should be able to eat as many calories as your body needs and still lose body fat. You can do this by eating the right foods for your body. More often the foods that we eat can be heavily processed and contain hidden fats, sugars and salt. Greater awareness of what we are putting into our mouths is essential.

When deciding on an eating programme for fat loss it is essential to realize that no single diet works for everyone. (In fact in the long-term diets work for no one!) At the moment diets and food advice tend to be general, when it is important to address individual needs. Some people need more carbohydrate, others more protein. Food can affect us in different ways: some people need to avoid certain

> If you consume too much food and you are inactive then you are going to be overweight!

foods, others to eat more. We are all made up differently, we all process food differently. That means paying attention to your own metabolic needs – what you eat, when you eat, how you eat. You need to train your body as to what works for you. (*see* chapter 5, p. 100, for further advice.)

Energy Out

We are an incredibly inactive nation that essentially needs to get off its backside. A British Heart Foundation survey revealed that only 37 per cent of men and 25 per cent of women are moderately active for the recommended 30 minutes five times a week. Now, a simple truism: if you consume too much food and you are inactive then you are going to be overweight. And not only will you become overweight you will also lose strength and tone in your muscles, your internal organs could suffer and your heart, circulatory system and digestive system may work less efficiently. Inactivity can also lessen your bone density, leading to conditions such as osteoporosis. In short, to become slimmer you need to be consistently active (*see* the exercises in chapter 6, p. 124).

Genetics

It is acknowledged that if one parent or both of your parents is or are obese or overweight then the likelihood is increased that you will be too. But, although body type is inherited, you cannot blame your parents for the amount of weight you carry. Although the number of fat cells in your body has been laid down genetically, the amount of fat they hold is down to you and your lifestyle. It may be that you have also inherited or learned your parents' eating habits as well. Your parents are a good guide as to what and what not to do – as the case may be.

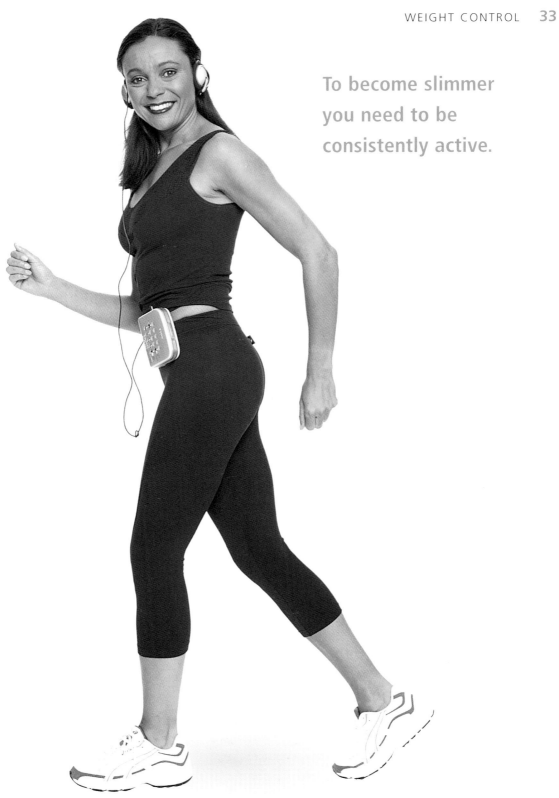

To become slimmer
you need to be
consistently active.

Age

Children, on the whole, do not become overweight unless they are completely inactive or utterly overfed. Hormones influence your adolescent body shape, and by your mid-teens genetics and lifestyle have dictated the number and condition of your fat cells. Your metabolic rate reaches its peak at the age of 20 and declines thereafter; around 30 you start to lose muscle mass and increase body fat; as you become older and your metabolism continues to slow down, you continue to gain weight. However, we do not need to allow this to happen. By moderating your eating patterns, taking regular exercise and remaining active you can maintain and increase your muscle mass and keep your weight under control as you get older.

Much interesting research has been carried out on the population of the Japanese island of Okinawa. This culture has the greatest number of centenarian and super-centenarians (people aged 110-plus!) on this earth. These people have remarkably low levels of body fat and remain physically active well into their eighties and nineties. There are a number of reasons for this, but foremost among them is that Okinawans habitually eat until they are not quite full – and no more – and are fully active throughout their lives.

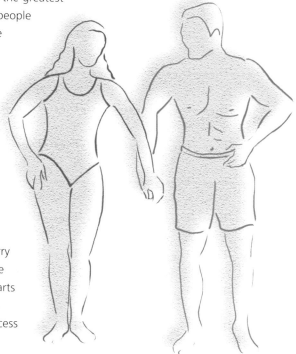

Women tend to hold their excess fat around their hips, thighs and bottom.

Gender

Female hormones mean that women typically carry more body fat than man. This hormonal influence also results in fat being distributed to different parts of the body at different points during a woman's lifetime. For example, most women hold their excess

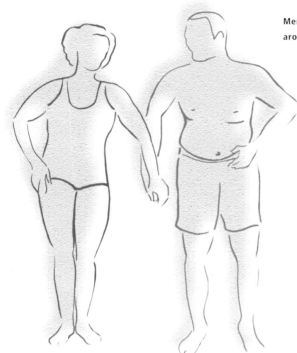

Men tend to put on weight around their upper body.

fat on the hips, thighs and bottom. But menopause can cause this fat to be redistributed around the middle. Men, on the other hand, tend to put on weight around their upper body and middle (male fat distribution is dictated by the anabolic hormones produced by the adrenal glands). Research has suggested that hip and thigh fat are harder to shift and that abdominal fat is easier to get rid of. Worth bearing in mind, however, is the fact that excess abdominal fat can predispose you to certain health problems, including cardiovascular disease, diabetes and apple-shaped obesity.

Environment

We have already seen how our eating is driven and encouraged by the availability and marketing of food; in other words, by our consumerist society. Our social environment (which has also been alluded to) also exerts an extremely significant influence on our eating behaviour. As children our minds are moulded by the behaviour of our parents – what they say explicitly and how they act – and by the messages – in the broadest sense – we take in from the world around us. So, some more truisms: if you live in a calm environment on a simple, natural, healthy diet you are less likely to be troubled by your weight; however, if your environment is stressful or makes you unhappy, you are more likely to turn to quick fixes to alleviate hunger and to fast-food for relief from your high-pressure life. It is this type of living that causes people to develop disordered eating patterns.

Now, our environment is a 'doing' one rather than a 'being' one: there is great pressure on us to do, to achieve, to succeed. And when that pressure stresses us out one of the body's inbuilt mechanism kicks in: the fight-or-flight response. This is a primitive reflex to perceived danger. To take a simple example, our distant ancestors, confronted by a predator, would have to run from it or confront it; and the fight-or-flight response prepares you for either by, among other things, increasing the heart rate and the amount of blood pumped to the muscles. But today's dangers are the stresses caused by overwork, perhaps by relationship or family problems or financial worries, and fight and flight are rarely realistic options – instead the body looks for other ways of coping with the stress, and one way of doing so is by overeating. But essentially – and this is a very important point – it is how we deal with that stress, how we perceive it, that determines our physiological reaction.

Disease

Experts say that in a few cases obesity is a result of trauma affecting the appetite-regulating centres in the brain. But for the most part obesity is more definitely attributed to lifestyle – to overeating and disordered eating habits. Obesity has also been linked to other factors. Having a poorly functioning thyroid can also cause weight gain. Excess weight will certainly predispose you to a number of diseases: heart disease, diabetes, osteoarthritis, high blood pressure and Syndrome X (a cluster of related disorders including the inability to properly deal with dietary carbohydrates and sugars, and high blood pressure). And being overweight may exacerbate conditions such as polycistic ovarian syndrome and other hormonal disturbances.

The best slimming strategy lies within – you are the only person who can give you a 100 per cent guarantee.

Psychological

You may have spent a lot of time addressing your weight but without any material success. This may be because you focused on external resources (the latest bit of kit or diet that promised to get you slim) or relied on others to help and tell you how to control your weight. But now a new trend is emerging that addresses the psychological aspects of weight management. This approach is a holistic one, regarding an individual as the sum total of their experience rather than focusing on just the physical body. In the past we have concentrated on 'what to do'; now we are addressing 'how to be'.

Past prejudice suggests that to consider the psychological aspect of something – anything – is to imply that there is something wrong with you; the language of self-exploration has been dismissed as psychobabble. But what can possibly be wrong with exploring your experience in order to realize your full potential and be the best you can be; and so what if emotions pop up that need to be confronted. It is now a well-established fact that mind and body act as one: every thought we think, every feeling we feel produces a chemical change in our body. Negative emotional states can have a very damaging effect on us physically. And knowing this, surely it is better to work on achieving emotional balance, controlling and managing emotions in a positive way rather than suppressing them with negative behaviours such as overeating. It is by understanding our emotions that we learn about ourselves and enable ourselves to become so much stronger. As you explore your experience you will discover the incredible internal resources you have within you and learn how to make use of them to come up with strategies for success – and not only in weight control.

I am not talking about a quick fix here. It may take some time for change to take place. But how long is up to you and your level of commitment to change. You may come up against obstacles or resistance but that's all they are – and they can be overcome. Make your first positive change and call your obstacles 'challenges' instead.

If you always do what you have always
done you will always get the same result.

It's time now to begin the process of training your mind as well as your body, setting yourself achievable weight management goals. It's time now to think yourself trim from the inside out as well as the outside in.

You can begin the process of thinking yourself trim by keeping a journal that will act as a complete record of your relationship with food. Design your journal so as to make a note of your past and present experience and what you desire for the future. The purpose of the journal is to help you commit yourself to the process of exploration and change.

On the front page of your journal draw up a contract to yourself that will confirm and record your commitment. Then get a friend to read and sign the contract; someone who you can discuss the process with as you go along to further enhance your motivation and verify the changes that are taking place.

The Think Yourself Trim Contract

I .... commit to fully explore my relationship

with food and dieting. I undertake to make the changes

that are necessary to achieve my trim, natural body weight.

Signed ....

Countersigned ....

Write a list of everything you have tried to do so far to control your weight. Put them into columns headed 'Successful' and 'Unsuccessful'. And if you did lose weight, was the loss short term or long term? Are you still following the same programmes?

What has weight control meant to you physically, mentally, emotionally? Jot down your thoughts. If you continue with your current methods of losing weight what do you think the result will be.

If you always do what you have always done you will always get the same result. If you have not had much success at weight management in the past maybe now is the time to do something different. Keep reading.

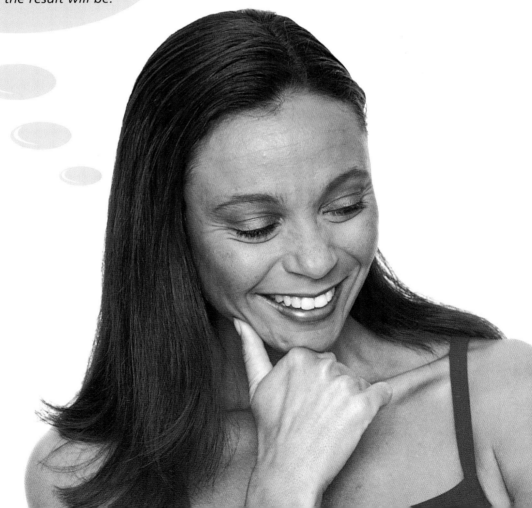

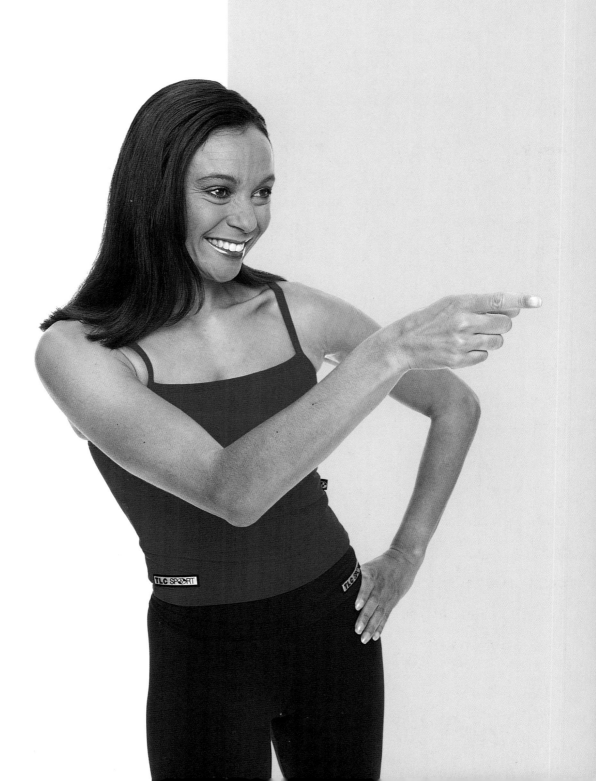

Chapter 3

The Workings of Your Mind

You are a human information-processing system made up of neural networks in every part of your body. Your brain has been likened to a computer. This magnificent organ – as big as a coconut, walnut shaped, its colour a lighter shade of mushroom, with the density of chilled butter! – weighs around 1.3 kg (3 lbs) and contains around 1,000,000,000,000 individual neurones. These neurones have been described as the circuits of the computer. But, in fact, such is the capacity of the human brain that the biggest computer in the world has nothing to equal the brain's billions of connections and neurones and its potential. Despite our technological advances we are unable to create anything to match it.

The Workings of Your Mind

The brain has two hemispheres: left and right. The left brain is 'masculine'; it is logical, analytical and time sensitive and responsible for language and intellect; it is associated with the conscious mind. It is thought that most people are left-brain dominant. The right brain is 'feminine'; it is emotional, artistic, creative, dreamy, holistic and associated with the subconscious mind. Both right and left brains are joined together by a fibrous band called the corpus callosum. This band conveys a continuous dialogue between the two hemispheres, so that they are interrelated in their working. The mind functions on two levels: the conscious mind at 10 per cent, the unconscious mind at 90 per cent.

Your Conscious Mind

Your conscious mind is your contact with reality in the waking state; it is characterized by awareness. We take in information through our senses: sight, sound, smell, taste and feeling, and it is thought that every second we have the capacity to take in huge amounts of information. To avoid sensory overload the information is filtered and deleted so that the information we are conscious of at any given moment is typically seven – plus or minus two bits of information. In other words, we can pay attention to between only five and nine things at a time – the phone ringing, the baby crying, the news on TV, the remark of our spouse, the kettle boiling … The conscious mind is a filtering service: if we didn't have it the result would be sensory overload – in other words, we would go nuts!

The information taken in is sorted, analysed, evaluated and judged. It is then presented to the subconscious part of your mind to be stored in the memory, waiting there to be brought back to consciousness when needed. The conscious mind is the goal setter, it makes decisions and directs your actions and it exercises the power of choice.

The mind functions on two levels: the conscious mind at 10 per cent, the unconscious mind at 90 per cent.

The brain has two hemispheres: left and right. The left brain is logical and analytical and the right brain is artistic and creative.

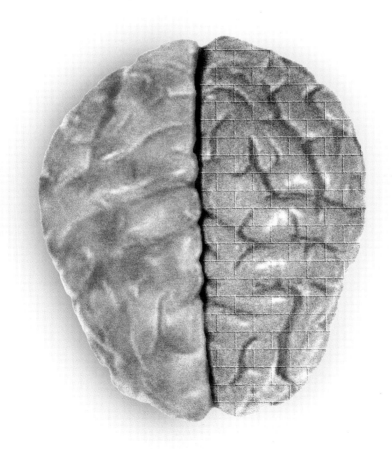

Look around you and see how much information you can take in at any point. See if you become more aware of the sights, smells, sounds, taste, and feelings around you by focusing on individual items. You will find that, even if you concentrate, you will be able to consciously register only a limited amount of information.

Self-awareness

The conscious mind is the part of you that is self-aware. One of its jobs is to establish the reality of the self. In other words we automatically act out the self that we believe ourselves to be. Consider this question: how do you know that you exist? Answer, because you are aware. You are aware of your body and its surroundings. Being aware confirms that the conscious mind is present and active.

How aware of your current eating patterns are you?

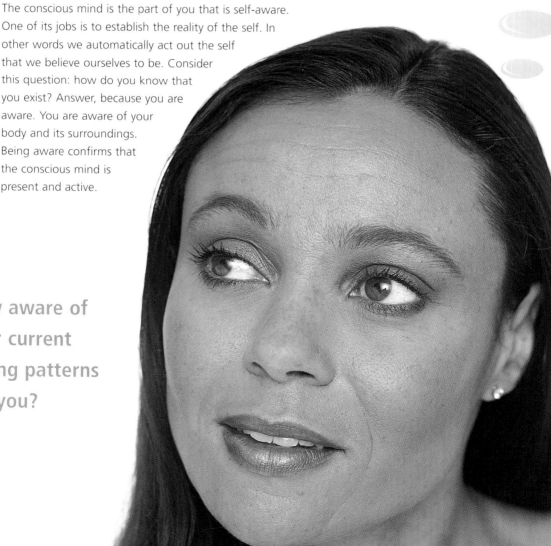

'It is the conscious mind that is the executive part of your total being. It is your conscious mind that makes decisions and translates them into action.' M. Scott Peck, *The Road Less Travelled*

QUESTIONNAIRE

Do any of the following behaviour patterns sound familiar?
Tick those that do.

- 'I start a diet on Monday but by Wednesday it's all gone wrong.'
- 'I can't just have one chocolate – I have to have the whole box.'
- 'I struggle with my weight all the time.'
- 'I cannot live without my bathroom scales.'
- 'Food rules my life.'
- 'I'm always on a diet.'
- 'I can't stop picking at food.'
- 'I get unbelievable cravings for certain foods.'
- 'I eat on the run.'
- 'I never know when to stop eating.'
- 'I am no longer as active as I used to be.'
- 'I don't have time to exercise.'
- 'I do not have any will-power where food is concerned.'
- 'I have been on so many diets but I just seem to get fatter and fatter.'
- 'I eat properly in front of other people but when I go home I have loads of goodies.'
- 'My husband comes home late so I help myself to the children's leftovers.'
- 'Waste not, want not.'
- 'I am never honest with myself about what I really eat.'
- 'I am fine during the day but I can't wait to get home at night to eat what I want.'
- Are there any others that you could add?

Make a committed decision now to begin to explore and focus on and become more consciously aware of the eating patterns that really need your attention, particularly the ones you have circled. Begin to notice what you eat, how you eat, how much food is on your plate; and your general attitude and behaviour towards food. Take a few minutes every day to jot down your experiences. (Preferably just after eating when it is fresh in your mind.)

As you look over your answers give yourself some feedback. Are you now more aware of any patterns that you may have with food? Clearly the more ticks you have made the more important it is that you address these areas. Are there some behaviours or patterns that appear more problematic than others? Circle those that seem to stick out.

Those eating patterns that you have just ticked are your behaviours, the result of what you think and feel. It is as result of these behaviours that you may carry excess weight on your body. You may find that you are not aware of some of those behaviours while you are actually doing them or at least you weren't giving them much conscious thought at the time. Often it may seem like you are running on automatic pilot. This is because although it may seem on the surface that the conscious mind is in charge, in fact the conscious mind is very much under the control of your subconscious.

Some of you are probably saying 'Yes, yes, I hear all this and I'm aware of what I do yet I just don't seem to have the will-power to do anything about it.' Another function of the conscious mind is to impose its will-power to set the direction towards a given goal; but it is often not effective in the long term without the agreement and support of the subconscious mind. Conscious will-power is powerless to make changes on its own. This is because the harder you have to try to do something the less chance you have of accomplishing it. You may reason with yourself that you should not eat that last chocolate éclair but somehow it still ends up in

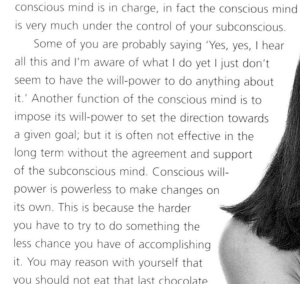

your mouth. On the whole, when you try to reason yourself out of eating you are setting yourself up for failure – you cannot compete with the desires of the subconscious mind.

It is also very important to realize that your brain responds to the suggestions that you give it but deletes the negatives. So if you say to yourself, 'I must not have an extra helping of pudding. I really must not have it', what do you think is likely to happen? Delete the nots and you have the answer. You are likely to be focusing on, and bringing about, the very thing you don't want.

We base our decisions on the strengths of our desires, and the desires of your subconscious mind are far stronger than those of your conscious mind. Although the conscious mind has the ability to reason it cannot carry through a decision until the subconscious mind agrees and directs its energy towards that goal. No amount of will-power will override the subconscious – emotion is more powerful than reason!

Explore
your experience with will-power. In
what areas of your life has will-power worked for
you? In what areas has it not worked? What is the difference
between these last two questions. How does your will-power affect
your experience with food? What is your behaviour as a result of
restricting yourself from enjoying food? Can you say no to those nibbles
at parties? How long do diets last for you? Can you resist that last
cream bun on the plate even though you are full,
or can you leave food on your plate
when you don't need it?

Write
your answers in your
journal.

You may now be thinking, 'What's the point if will-power doesn't work all of the time.' (And quite possibly if you are a veteran dieter you are already aware that in the long term will-power alone doesn't work.) Well, quite right! Clearly there is no point in putting yourself through the discomfort that is involved in losing weight through using conscious will power alone. Do not despair – the mind has the most enormous capacity for change. You can control your eating behaviour by harnessing your conscious will-power to the desire of the subconscious and directing both towards the common goal of a trimmer you. You just need to find out how.

Linking Mind to Body

It is essential that you realize that what you think – positive or negative – has a powerful effect on you physically, right down to the cellular level. If you overeat you are most likely to wear the result of your overindulgence on your body in the form of excess fat. If you eat poor-quality foods you are likely to be affected mentally and physically, because your mind and body aren't getting the nourishment they require. If you allow the bathroom scales to rule your life there are going to be times when you jump on them full of hope only for those hopes to be dashed. You will probably give up, frustrated and disheartened, whatever diet or exercise programme you are on and head straight for the biscuit bin. The result? The very thing you want to avoid. What you do has an effect on your physical body and the way you feel about yourself, how you think and what you do.

*Stand
in front of the mirror in your
underwear or stark naked. Take a good look at
your body, see the effects of your past behaviour on
your body. Begin by taking your awareness to your overall
body shape. Be aware of your posture. Look at the shape
of your body, its contours. Take that awareness to your
muscle tone; feel your muscles if you wish.*

*Now
focus on what covers that muscle. Be
aware of the amount of fat you have on your body,
really look at it. Does that fat seem to be concentrated
in one particular place - around your middle, bottom or
thighs, across your shoulders even? Take hold of it if you
want to. Can you pinch more than an inch of fat? Is it soft or
hard? Now take your attention to your skin, its colour,
texture, tone. Look again at your overall body shape
and then step back from the mirror.*

Awareness is the key to all change.

Sorry, that may have been a little cruel of me. Or perhaps that's negative thinking on my part: you were really giving yourself praise and fully appreciating your fine form? Weren't you?

Often we choose not to be aware of ourselves to avoid what we don't want to see especially if we don't feel good about ourselves; or we don't want to address or modify our behaviour because there are so many other things to occupy us. But essentially we are not aware of many aspects of ourselves until we take the time to consider them consciously. Sometimes people are simply not aware of how they abuse their bodies with their eating patterns. The abuse does not just result in what you see on the outside, it also affects you mentally and emotionally. Quite often people are simply not connected to their bodies.

I remember an obese client who came to see me who insisted that she didn't feel fat and went about life quite happily. She didn't have any full-length mirrors in her house, but she would sometimes get a shock when she caught her reflection in a shop window. She then became very much aware that she was very overweight, which resulted in feelings of shame and humiliation. And it was only when this was brought to consciousness and she made the connection between mind and body that she felt compelled to do something about it.

Your conscious mind allows you to discriminate between what is desirable and what is not. These values are based on the information that has been fed into your subconscious and formed the beliefs you hold about yourself and food. As you performed that last exercise you may have found yourself making some tough value judgements about your body. Some of them perhaps quite unjustified. However, if you really want to lose weight you need to take that step in increasing your awareness.

The Subconscious Mind

The subconscious mind is the part of you that functions outside of your current awareness. It also accomplishes more and is more powerful than the conscious mind. The subconscious is made up of all those mental processes that operate on a day-to-day basis without our knowledge. (Have you ever travelled from A to B without noticing how many bus stops or train stations you have passed, or driven to your destination and arrived with no recollection of what happened along the way? This is your subconscious mind at work.) But do not think that your conscious and unconscious minds are completely separate, they work together in an interrelated way. Your subconscious mind has been likened to a robot, relentlessly moving and steering towards the goals it is set.

If the conscious mind is the goal setter then the subconscious mind is the goal getter. Most people remain unaware of their subconscious minds and its incredible potential to enable them to reach their goals in life, a lack of awareness that can result in underachievement. Your subconscious mind works for you 24 hours a day, although it is only when you go to sleep – when you are unconscious – that your conscious mind recedes and your subconscious mind takes over. The subconscious holds our values, the criteria on which we base our judgements. It acts upon the ideas and suggestions presented to it by the conscious, reasoning mind. However, once an idea has been accepted by the subconscious it can be there for ever. For any change to take place you need to convince your subconscious. The subconscious mind is an untapped force right there inside of you waiting to do your will. Some people travel on a quest for answers that could easily be found by looking inwards for guidance. But a very important point: the subconscious mind does not discriminate between positive or negative thoughts, positive or negative ambitions.

Your subconscious mind needs to be controlled. Or it will control you, which is very much the case with many of us. It may control you because your conditioning has established certain beliefs and values in your

Look back at your life and jot down your experiences of the subconscious mind at work. Do you eat without being aware of it? Do you finish a meal and have no recollection of what happened while you were eating?

What are your thoughts about your unconscious processes? How do those processes that we have discussed so far rule your life? Do you feel ruled by your subconscious desires? What can you do to make yourself more conscious of what you eat?

Make a decision to notice or get a friend or a member of the family to let you know when you are unconsciously making decisions with food. In other words, reaching for the biscuit tin.

subconscious: for example, 'My parents ate a lot, so will I', 'Eating has always made me happy in the past.' So you can understand why your eating patterns appear to be beyond your control or why you seem to eat without thinking. And once an eating pattern is accepted by the subconscious it becomes hard to change. However, we have resources within us to make changes at a subconscious level. You can develop a new awareness of self by getting in touch with that greater part of yourself that has been controlled by others or by circumstance. You can steer your mind to get *you* to where you want to go.

Although we have free will to do anything we want, our decisions are based on the strengths of our desires, and those desires originate in our subconscious mind. So, you are overweight and make the decision to go on a diet, yet you find it difficult to follow through and it all ends in failure. You have decided something consciously but are unable to accept it subconsciously – the two parts of your mind are not in agreement.

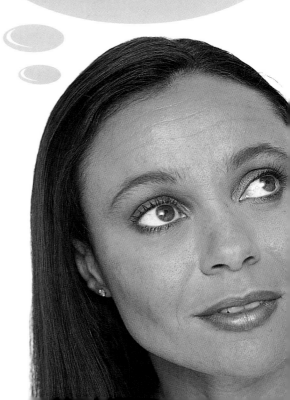

Change your habits, behaviour, emotions
and self-image.

 ## A Storer of Information

Your subconscious mind contains all your life's experiences both positive
and negative. You take in information from the outside world and store it
in the subconscious memory banks ready to be recalled when it is needed.
Your whole relationship with food, which includes your food habits, your
food beliefs, your food behaviour, has been stored in your mind.

The automatic personality traits that we have today develop during our
formative years, laying the foundations on which we have built our lives.
When we are very young – until our critical faculties began to develop
around the age of five or six – our brain is like a sponge, absorbing
everything around us. Our parents are our first 'hypnotherapists'. During
those early years we accept everything that we are told, unable to
discriminate between ideas that are helpful or detrimental.

You are likely to have picked up eating patterns from your parents and
accepted unquestioningly the food that was given to you. If you were
brought up on processed food you are likely to be perfectly happy with
processed food later in life; if you were brought up on organic food you
are more likely to want to eat organic food throughout your life. Your eating
experience at the table might have been relaxed, and you may have been
encouraged to eat slowly and comfortably. If you came from a large family
you might have had to fight for the last piece of bread. Family meals may
have been fun or fraught with tension. Whatever your experience, it is in
those formative years that most behaviours are established.

For some people food is a means to an end – fuel to get you through
the day; for others eating is in itself a pleasurable experience. In those
formative years we learn to eat food for reasons other than hunger. We
discover that having something in our mouths is an immensely comforting
experience. Babies suckle on their mothers' breasts, and small children are
given pacifiers or pieces of cloth as they grow older; children only have to
yell and they are given food to comfort them (or simply to shut them up).
We are cajoled into eating later in life whether we are hungry or not

because our parents worry that we aren't eating enough. Later we are told to finish the food on our plate, to think of the starving in other parts of the world. We are given food to reward us for being good and deprived of it for being bad. (If you have children, are all these familiar? Were you brought up in the same way?) And all this is stored in the computer-like mind.

Often when you try to make changes as adults they are contrary to the experiences stored in your memory. Hence change is not always easy. Your memories are stored as images, sounds, smells, tastes, sensations, and it is time now to recapture them as you explore your past relationship with food.

Sit in a comfortable position in which you can completely relax; have your journal ready to note your experience. Take ten deep breaths, inhaling for a count of four and exhaling for a count of six. Pick one of the simple statements that you circled on the questionnaire. And ask yourself, 'Where did I learn that?' Now focus on the last time you did this and then allow your mind to take you back in time to the original experience. Fully explore that experience. See the experience from an observer's position – so that you are looking on at the situation and you are detached emotionally.

What can you learn from this experience? Imagine the observer is also the advisor. What advice might you give to the younger you that would make a difference today? What could you do instead? Think of two new behaviours to take the place of the old one.

Your subconscious mind responds to real and imaginary experiences.

For example, I have two memories. The first memory that comes to mind is when I became a mother. I constantly worried that my son was not eating enough. He was a happy baby but didn't seem to want to eat much, especially in the evening. He would refuse to eat the food that I had carefully prepared for him and would never finish the food on his plate. It was time for a familiar trick. I would pretend that the spoon was an aeroplane whizzing through the air. My son would start to laugh as it came nearer and nearer, and before he realized or could refuse, it was in his mouth. It was a great game, but alas not for long. That bright, intelligent little boy soon cottoned on and kept his mouth firmly shut.

What did I learn? That he simply wasn't hungry and I was in fact overfeeding him. It was my problem and it was an unjustified worry that he was not getting enough. He was given a number of bottles throughout the day and had cereal for breakfast and a healthy lunch as well as crusts to chew on. If I were in that situation today I would trust that he knew what his body needed. He would let me know when he was hungry. So, two new behaviours: I would relax more, I would also learn to tune in to my son's behaviour so that I recognized the signs of real hunger.

The second memory is of Sunday lunch at the family table. There were four children in my family and my parents had a waste-not mentality and didn't like to see food left on the plate. On Sundays we were treated to the West Indian dish of ackee and salt fish followed by rice and gungu peas and roast lamb and vegetables. More than anything I wanted to please my father by eating the food and avoiding waste, and I used to eat to bursting point, having second and even third helpings so that I could hardly move afterwards.

It is great to identify with your origins and to be open to exotic foods, but today I know that in wanting to please somebody else I was eating far more than was good for me. If I had continued to eat in that way – if my parents hadn't realized what was happening – I would soon have begun to pile on the pounds.

Imagination is more powerful than reason.

The two new behaviours I would put in place would be to put only a certain amount of food on my plate; and to savour and enjoy each delicious mouthful. It is, of course, not the quantity of food that counts, but the quality. And that would have pleased my father just as much. Now, if you ticked quite a few of the statements on the questionnaire, take the time to do this exercise with every one of them.

So, we have taken a trip down memory lane and you are now beginning see how you might have learned your current eating patterns. As you explored your experience you would have been aware that the memories came back to you not just as pictures, but with sounds and smells and more. Some of you would have remembered experiences more vividly than others. How vividly you remember a scene depends on the quality of the attention you give it.

Your Imagination

We are not born negative. We are born with positive, lively imaginations. As we grow older we may begin to suppress our imagination or experience may encourage us to use it negatively. Often what we accept as true is only a suggestion or an idea that we imagine to be true, and we begin to act out that perceived truth as if it were true. If the suggestions are positive then your thinking and beliefs about yourself will be positive and will empower you ('I can lose weight'). But if the suggestions are negative then the result is negative thinking and limiting beliefs that will prevent you from achieving success ('I'll never be as slim as I want to be').

For those of who are saying 'I have no imagination', well, that really isn't true. Everybody has an imagination, you just might have suppressed yours and that needs to be addressed, because we all draw on our imagination for problem-solving and creative inspiration. Dreams and dream-like states have inspired scientists and artists alike. Your imagination is most dominant when the conscious, reasoning mind is dormant. This is

Stand with your feet hip distance apart and your knees slightly soft. Take your right arm out at shoulder level. Focus your eyeline on your finger. Rotate your trunk and gently twist as far as you comfortably can. Now mark that point. Centre your body again. Now close your eyes and imagine yourself doing the same thing, but imagine that you can go beyond the point that you have just marked. As you imagine yourself turning further, allow your body to follow your mind – you should find that you can go a little further than you did a moment ago.

most likely to be when you go to bed at night and at those just-awake moments in the morning or when you completely switch off and relax. The exercise above shows the imagination at work.

Often you can do so much more than you think you can do. In the exercise above your imagination made it possible for you to go so much further than you thought you could. This amazing power can be applied to many areas of life, including creating a trimmer you.

Imagination and Your Weight

We create images in our minds all the time even though we are not aware that we do so. They can be positive or negative. The images we create are heavily influenced by the messages we give to ourselves and those given to us by others. Often the result of the messages from the outside world is pressure to conform and a fear of not being able to conform. Fear can fuel our imagination to work powerfully for us to achieve our goals. But sometimes we begin to use our imagination negatively, focusing on the problems and discomfort involved in losing weight and on how inadequate we are. So we find ourselves creating 'fat pictures' in our minds and worrying about being overweight and the food that we should avoid. This is very dangerous: the subconscious mind will accept these negative images and thoughts as the goals it has to work towards. We said earlier that the subconscious mind doesn't discriminate between positive and negative. If you believe that you are overweight, you are most likely to create images in your mind that support this belief – and your subconscious will provide the energy to work towards them. If you believe that you will fail to get trim, your subconscious will do its best to 'help' you fail. You get what you focus on. Focus on what you want to avoid and your subconscious mind will work to make it come true.

Relaxation and Your Imagination

Your imagination is at its most powerful when you are fully relaxed. And that doesn't mean just sitting down with a cup of tea or watching the telly. When you are deeply relaxed your mind is open to change and you can direct it to work towards your dreams. Through practice we can easily achieve these deeply relaxed states, and in fact we do so naturally when we daydream or in the moments before or after sleep. The conscious mind recedes and the subconscious mind comes to the fore. This shift in consciousness allows you direct access to the subconscious mind, and it is in this state that you can take control of and direct it.

Before doing any of the exercises in this book in which you use your imagination, prepare yourself with the exercise on the opposite page.

How does your imagination work for you – mostly positively or negatively? Make two columns in your journal and head them 'Positive' and 'Negative' and write down a few examples of both.

For example, I remember when I was a model desperately wanting to get a particular job. So I imagined how positive I was going to be at the audition, how I would respond to the photographer and clients and how I could persuade them that I was the best person for that job. I imagined being successful and getting the job. And guess what – I did just that.

But I also remember that I used to be very nervous about public speaking. I was always convinced that the audience was criticizing me. I imagined that I would dry up completely or forget what I was saying. And the result? I avoided speaking publicly unless I absolutely had to, and when I did I would dry up.

Now what do you imagine with regard to eating and the weight you hold on your body? Write down your experience.

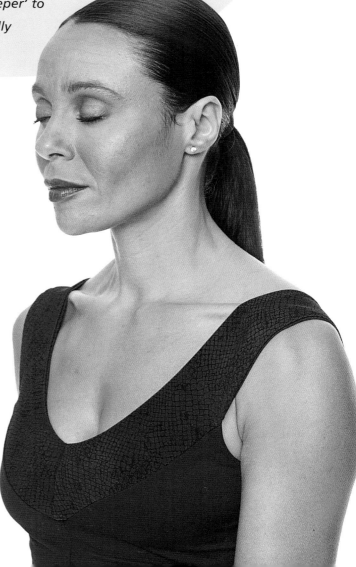

Make sure you will not be disturbed and that you are wearing comfortable clothing. Sit comfortably and take your attention to each muscle in your body. Tell each muscle to relax. Start from your feet and work you way up to the top of your head. Do this slowly and feel your muscles get heavy and relaxed. When you have reached the top of your head, imagine that you are at the top of a flight of stairs and count down from twenty to one. Breathe deeply between each step. When you reach the bottom step spend a few moments with your breathing, saying 'deeper and deeper' to yourself until you are fully relaxed.

Think of a time when your imagination worked really well for you. For example when you came up with a great idea or you created something you were really proud of. Relive the experience and as you think about it recall what you saw, heard and felt. Be aware of the colours of the experience – are they bright, light and clear? Remember the sounds – perhaps you heard laughter, a positive voice. Be aware of your feelings as you recapture this experience.

Now pick one of the statements that you ticked on the questionnaire. What would you rather imagine instead? For example, instead of 'I struggle with my weight all the time' tell yourself 'I am in control of my weight' and see it.

Focus on how you would rather imagine yourself to be. See yourself successfully losing weight. Now add the colour sounds and feelings from the previous, successful picture to this one. But make the picture even brighter, the tonality even more positive, the feel-good factor stronger and bigger. Create this image in full technicolor. Then open your eyes and come back into the room.

Programming Your Mind

The conscious mind can be likened to the captain of a ship planning his journey. The captain plots the course with much careful thought, pours over his maps and charts and then sets his compass to make sure he will get his ship safely to its destination. However, the ship won't get there without the fuel it needs. Your subconscious mind can be likened to the engine of the ship, providing energy and drive to power you on the course it has been given, to get you where you want to go in life.

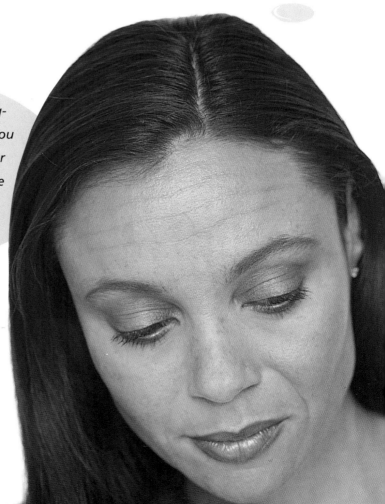

If you are having difficulty imagining what it will be like to be trim, think of somebody you know who is trim. Imagine stepping into their shoes. Act as they would. Imagine what you would see, hear, feel. Perhaps you'd see people looking at you admiringly, hear them telling you that you look great; you'd feel lighter (in every sense), happier and more confident about yourself. Again, let these feelings get bigger and bigger until they almost peak. Then lock them in with your non-dominant hand – make a fist. Those feelings will always be there for you, and you can call upon them whenever you need the motivation to become trimmer.

Imagine that you are having a mental spring-clean. Throw out any pictures in which you are fat or overweight or any images of your negative eating patterns. Now replace those pictures with positive images of you as you would rather be instead.

What your mind sees your body will do.

Think now of the people you know who have set targets in their lives. Were they successful or unsuccessful? Did they use positive or negative language to reach or not to reach their targets? What was it that made them successful or unsuccessful?

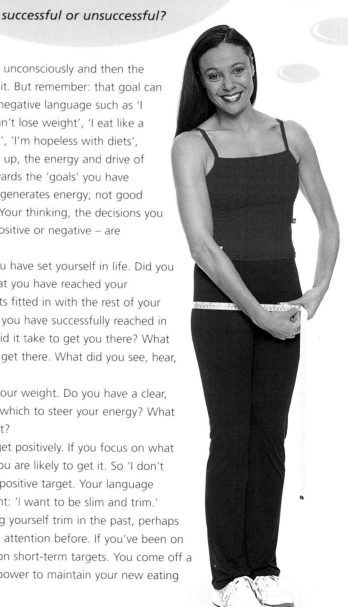

Human beings are naturally goal-oriented. We are target seekers. We set a goal either consciously or unconsciously and then the subconscious mind works towards it. But remember: that goal can be positive or negative. If you use negative language such as 'I keep trying not be so fat', 'I just can't lose weight', 'I eat like a pig', 'My hips and thighs are so fat', 'I'm hopeless with diets', and you create images to back this up, the energy and drive of your subconscious powers you towards the 'goals' you have programmed in. The subconscious generates energy; not good energy or bad energy, just energy. Your thinking, the decisions you make, your behaviour – whether positive or negative – are expressions of that energy.

Think about the targets that you have set yourself in life. Did you reach them? How do you know that you have reached your destination? How have these targets fitted in with the rest of your life? Think now of a specific target you have successfully reached in the past. What internal resources did it take to get you there? What did you say to yourself to help you get there. What did you see, hear, feel at the time?

Think of your experience with your weight. Do you have a clear, realistic, achievable target towards which to steer your energy? What will happen if you don't set a target?

Make sure you phrase your target positively. If you focus on what you don't want, just remember – you are likely to get it. So 'I don't want to be fat any longer' is not a positive target. Your language should reflect what it is you do want: 'I want to be slim and trim.'

If you've had difficulty imagining yourself trim in the past, perhaps you've never really given it your full attention before. If you've been on diets you may have been focusing on short-term targets. You come off a diet hoping that you have the will-power to maintain your new eating

Set yourself a realistic, specific target for an ideal body weight now.

patterns in the future. The problem is that the subconscious mind has been programmed to reach a long-term goal. Therefore, you reach your short-term goal and then revert back to old behaviours. All change begins at a subconscious level. Quick fixes don't work in the long term and may even be detrimental to your well-being. Make sure that your target is one that you can maintain in the future. We are talking about a stable bodyweight for life – permanent weight loss, not temporary.

To achieve this it is essential that you are aware of the language you use and the images you create (are they positive or negative?), and that you to begin to direct your powerful subconscious mind towards the goal of a trimmer you. Remember, if you are not the captain of your ship, or you are unclear

Sit back in your relaxed position and breathe deeply; count down slowly from twenty to one. Allow your mind to clear.

Create a clear image of your goal. See yourself as you wish to be: lean, fit, slim, full of energy and vitality. See your body at its ideal weight and in its ideal shape. Make the image as clear as you can, as colourful as you can. Add some sound. Imagine how you would like to feel. Make the picture perfect for you in every way. When you have the perfect blueprint, imagine that you are stepping into the picture. And fully associate into those feelings. Allow the feelings to get bigger and bigger and then when they peak take your non-dominant hand and make a fist.

Whenever you need to bring this picture back in the future you just have to make that fist. Now open your eyes and list at least ten benefits that achieving this target will bring to you.

Focus on a stable weight for life.

about your destination, or you allow others to set your course for you, then your subconscious mind will still release its energy to reach 'goals' that may be entirely self-destructive. Charles Tebetts, director of the Washington Hypnotherapy Institute, likened the subconscious mind to a gushing fire hose: 'In the hands of an able fireman it quenches a fire and saves lives and properties. But if it is let loose it can wreak havoc and cause a lot of damage.'

The Heart of Change

All change takes place at a subconscious level. The scripts that you give yourself (how, in other words, you talk to yourself) are your very own recommendations for action and directions to that powerful force within you. For any real change to take place, it therefore makes sense to examine the language you use – language that has its origins in what has been said to you in the past, in the thousands of hours of subconscious recordings that you store – and examine the results of using that language.

Think about the things you say to yourself. The messages that you are giving your subconscious mind. Especially when you are having a 'fat day'. Make a list of the negative comments that you make about your weight.

- 'I feel so fat.'
- 'I hate my fat thighs.'
- 'I must get rid of the dimples on my bum.'
- 'Yuck! Just look at my flabby arms.'

Now use the following guidelines to turn these comments into positives. The first thing you need to do is omit the negative words. So avoid 'can't', 'try', 'won't', 'don't', in fact any words that presuppose the possibility of failure. 'I will try to lose weight' presupposes that you may fail. 'I am no longer fat' tells the subconscious mind to focus on the fact of being fat. Your suggestions should be target-oriented and specific to what you want. They should speak of the benefits that achieving your target will bring: how much weight you are going to lose and any other specific details that may be useful.

'I am no longer fat' should be

- 'I am slim and trim in a healthy way.'

'I no longer binge' should be

- 'I eat in a calm and relaxed way.'

Give yourself no more than two or three specific suggestions to work on related to your target. And keep your language simple and direct – the subconscious responds as if it were a 10-year-old.

Be Realistic

This is where many people go astray. Often we set completely unrealistic targets for our minds to follow, but now is the time to get real. If yours is a square, stocky body shape you are never going to look like Kate Moss. You are more likely to have an 'athletic' shape when you are at your best. If you are a curvaceous pear shape don't trying to emulate an amazon with strong shoulders and tiny hips. It is essential that you accept your natural body shape. The more you try to be something you are not, the less likely you are to achieve your weight-loss goals. Your weight is linked to your self-image, and once you have accepted your natural body shape you can work to make it the best it can be.

You also need to be sure not to set yourself

a target of drastic weight loss, or, worse still, to lose a lot of weight two weeks before you go on holiday. Many people go on extreme diets because their target is to lose weight quickly. They achieve this but they put the weight back on just as quickly – and sometimes extra. The World Health Organization suggests that 2 lb (just under 1 kg) of fat is the most that can be lost per week. Set your main target and then work out how long it will realistically take you to get there.

The Present Tense

Your subconscious mind responds best to the present tense. So even though your target is set for the future, you must talk to yourself in the present tense. Even so, avoid saying 'I am much slimmer than before' otherwise your subconscious mind is likely to focus on what it knows you were like before: overweight (and unhappy). Say 'In the future I will be slim' and you will find yourself waiting till tomorrow for it to start working for you. Avoid confusion: speak in the here and now – 'Every day I am working towards my target of getting into my size-10 jeans. Every day I am aware of how much food is on my plate and I know to leave food uneaten when I am comfortable and satisfied.'

Set a Time Limit

Although your language should be phrased in the present tense, you need to set a specific time by which you will have achieved your target weight. Do your homework and find out how long it will take. And then set the target in your mind: 'By such and such a time I will have achieved my target weight.' You may then choose to set further smaller targets leading up to that point. This will give you markers to work to on the way, and every time you reach one you can give yourself a pat on the back and then keep going.

Action Language

Focus your language on action rather than ability. Your subconscious will respond to 'I am getting slimmer every day' rather than 'I have the ability to lose weight.' Focus on what you will be doing to lose weight. 'I make an appointment with myself every day to exercise at the gym', 'I always take the stairs when I can', 'I sit down at the table and take the time to eat slowly and enjoy my lunch.'

Motivation

The subconscious mind is the seat of the emotions, and the more positive, motivational and enthusiastic your language is the more it is likely to respond. Give powerful emotional descriptions to your subconscious. I know this won't come easily to some people but don't worry, you won't get a big head. Go for it.

'I love the way that I look. I feel gorgeous. Every time I look in the mirror I am so proud that I am reaching my target weight. I have a strong desire to eat only foods that are good for my body. I am thrilled to be getting closer and closer to my ideal weight every day. My body feels sexier and sexier as I get fitter and fitter.'

Repetition

Repeat your positive affirmations for at least five minutes in the morning and in the evening and as often as you can at other times. Repeat the affirmations even if you feel resistant towards them (after all, if you really did believe 'I am slim' you wouldn't need to say it – but saying it will help it come true). Keep on saying them; act as if they were true; say them with feeling and passion. Visualize them as often as you can. The more you are exposed to an idea, the more likely you are to believe it. Focus on the benefits to come as your subconscious mind gets the message and works towards your goals. They say it takes 21 days to make a new habit permanent so it's important to keep reinforcing the idea.

Think of your target weight. And now think of the negative suggestions you have given yourself in the past. How can you turn them around so that they are positive and focused on your target? Write them down.

Make a committed decision to be aware of the language you use and learn to stop when you find yourself being negative. Take a deep breath. Replace the negative message with a positive message instead. Be patient as you learn to change your language – it takes time and practice.

Now as you look at your new suggestions. Visualize yourself following them through positively and confidently. Act out the suggestions and believe in them 100 per cent. I promise it will make a difference.

Involuntary Functions

Your subconscious mind is responsible for all the involuntary functions of your body. Think for a moment about your body and your internal organs – your digestive system, respiratory system, endocrine system, your reproductive and elimination systems. How is it that they work? How is that we blink without even being aware of it. Something has to be controlling all of those processes, and that something is your subconscious mind.

The hypothalamus is the part of the brain that regulates and controls the involuntary functions. It is situated in the midbrain, weighs about 14 g (or half an ounce) and is the size of a five-pence piece. This powerful gland also governs the mechanism that regulates your appetite and tells you when you are hungry and when you are satiated. It also lets you know when you are over-full. The hypothalamus plays a part in your emotional state, which explains why the emotions and food appear to be linked.

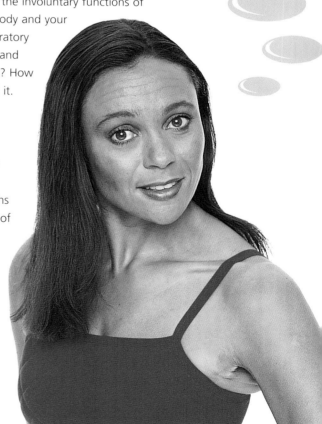

The appetite-control mechanism has an enormous effect on your body. When it functions well and normally you find both body and mind in balance. You know when you are hungry; you know when you are comfortably full. You are able to maintain a healthy bodyweight. But when the appetite-control mechanism is dysfunctional both physical and mental imbalances occur. Being overweight can be considered the result of a disordered appetite-control mechanism and poor nutrition. Dieting can cause much of this dysfunction; other factors are the way we manage and control our eating patterns and most importantly our eating behaviours.

I mentioned before that being overweight is the result of an abnormal environment. We live in a society where food is abundant and it is comforting to know that we will not go hungry. But what we must question is the quality of the food. It is of course impossible to compete with Mother Nature, but in the name of consumerism, we find shops full of foods packed with additives, preservatives, colourings and taste enhancers. It seems that rather than giving us the nutrition we need, these foods have had an adverse affect on both our minds and bodies, creating nutritional deficiencies, food cravings, disordered appetite-control mechanisms and metabolic weaknesses that can result in, among other things, diabetes, obesity, heart disease and mental and emotional disorders such as depression. On top of this, the way we manage and control our eating is not in harmony with nature.

So how can we get our bodies to function the way they should? And what would be the benefits of doing so? The benefits would be metabolic balance in the body, which would allow you to achieve your natural bodyweight; and a more nutritionally balanced mind and body. You have already addressed many of the mental aspects of your eating experience. Now it is time to train your body to get back in touch with its natural mechanisms, restoring the appetite-control mechanism so that it functions optimally. You can do this by further focusing your mind to train your body to know when you are hungry and when you are full. You can also do this by providing your body with optimum nutrition – in other words,

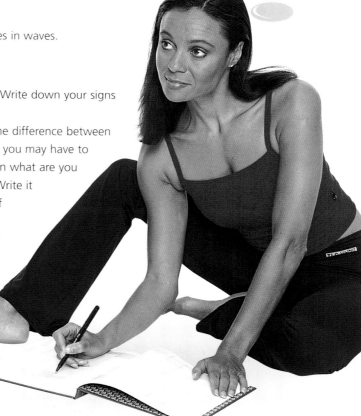

Ask yourself the following questions:
Do you only eat when you are hungry?
Do you wait until you are starving and then binge?
Do you eat before you get hungry?
Do you eat with others for the sake of it?
When was the last time that you felt really hungry?
Are there sensory triggers that set off feelings of hunger?

feeding your cells with nothing less than the best. The goal is an eating programme that is in harmony with your biology.

What does hunger feel like to you? How do you know when you are hungry? Here are some of the common hunger signals:

- A rumbling in your stomach
- Irritability
- Slight headache
- Difficulty concentrating
- A gnawing feeling that comes in waves.
- Slight restlessness
- Low energy and cravings

How many of these are familiar? Write down your signs of hunger in your journal.

Make a decision to learn to tell the difference between real hunger and any other urges that you may have to eat. If you are not feeling hungry then what are you feeling? Is it emotional or habitual? Write it down. And find an alternative way of satisfying that feeling.

This exercise should be done only when you can give it your full attention without worrying about other commitments and time restraints. So choose a weekend when you have the time to really focus.

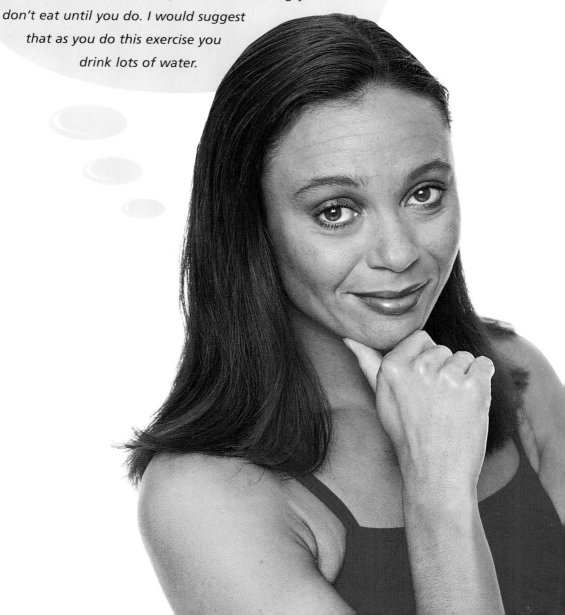

Commit today to eating only when you are hungry – and this does not mean starving yourself. If you try to deny your hunger it will keep coming back until you do something about it. If you don't feel hungry then don't eat until you do. I would suggest that as you do this exercise you drink lots of water.

Sit back and work through your body telling every muscle to relax. Count down from twenty to one and focus on your breathing as you do so.

Imagine a dial that represents your appetite-control centre. Give it a colour then number it one to ten: one to four being 'not very hungry'; five to seven being 'hungry'; eight to ten being 'famished'. Currently, what number does the dial have to point to before you eat? Just allow the number to come up in your mind.

Is your setting out of the normal hunger range – too high or too low? Use your imagination to reset the dial to the right number for you to eat at. Make a committed decision to go inside your mind every day and set this dial until you begin to feel the signs of real hunger and you know it is time to eat.

When you eat, eat until you feel satisfied, until you get a comfortable feeling in your stomach – not too full, not too empty. If you're not sure how this should feel, eat until you imagine that you have had the right amount. If you no longer feel hungry, stop eating. You can do this by paying attention to your eating experience. Eat your food slowly. Give it the full attention it deserves. Smell it, taste every mouthful, be aware of the texture, the temperature, the taste of the food. Then allow your body to give you the signal that it has had enough.

The above exercise is one I use with all my weight-loss clients. It has been adapted from an exercise devised by the Atkinson Ball College of Hypnosis.

Only eat when you are physically hungry and stop eating when you feel satisfied.

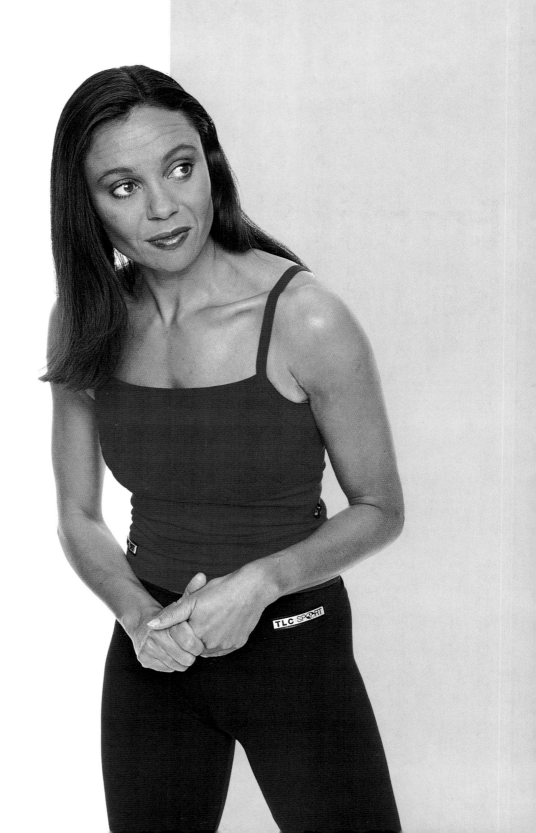

Chapter 4

Emotions and Habits

It has been said that that the subconscious mind is the seat of our emotions. We think of emotions as feelings but that is not the full picture. Essentially our emotions are a set of survival mechanisms that warn us of danger and help us move towards things that benefit us. They tell us when to run, when to laugh, when to get angry, when to relax. Emotions have been likened to colours: there are primary emotions and then as you mix those primary emotions you get a wide range of shadings each with its own label. The primary emotions are fear, anger, love and disgust.

Emotions and Habits

Emotions begin with an internal or an external stimulus. Other labels for emotional states – calm, helpless, annoyed, irritated, anxious, excited, depressed, curious, alert, guilty, joy, gratitude, resentment, sadness, contentment, jealously, shame etc. Once the mind perceives that a situation calls for an emotional response it sends a signal to the brain. The brain responds by sending messages to the body and then the body acts accordingly.

Our emotional states change from moment to moment depending on what we are thinking at the time. And emotions just seem to happen: it's impossible to catch them in the act. Try to control them at a conscious level and you are likely to get into trouble. Emotions are powerful things and they will always override reason.

Emotional Eating

Eating can be an immensely enjoyable experience. Human nature is very much influenced by what is painful and what is pleasurable. Sometimes we eat for pleasure as a way of dealing with the trials and tribulations of life that cause us pain or stress us out. Those trials and tribulations are often a result of living in today's high-pressured society and with the demands it places on us and that we place on ourselves.

I said above that our emotions tell us how to respond to a given situation. But in today's society we cannot (always) scream and shout when we are angry or run for the hills when we are frightened. We have to deal with stress in a different way. In a society that values and rewards excellence and perfection, food has become for some the quick fix, the sensory thrill, the few moments of gratification that reset the balance of our stressful lives. We have learned to cope with life by manipulating our emotions with food, and the result is eating patterns that can be described only as unnatural and disordered. We have also learned to feel deprived when we can't have those perceived treats. Yet all we are deprived of in the long-term is happiness, as our fast-food fixes leave us overweight and miserable and lacking the confidence and ambition to reach our goals in life.

Being overweight or having disordered eating patterns are very much symptoms of imbalance in some area of the mind or body. It is commonly acknowledged that to address a symptom is to look no further than the tip of the iceberg, to take nothing more than a surface view. The problem with a diet – and diet culture – is that it deals with the symptom and not the cause, which is why it is rarely successful in the long term. When it comes to addressing the causes of weight problems we find that they are simmering below the surface and are not obvious.

What we all normally do is recreate the environment of our home life in our mind and we carry this with us through life. So when we lack belief in ourselves or our abilities, when we feel scared or insecure we overeat to comfort ourselves. When we feel threatened we put on weight to protect ourselves. When we feel lonely we fill the void by eating. When we have coped with a stressful day we reward ourselves with food.

Case studies

COMFORT EATING

- Subject: an obese 49-year-old who yo-yo diets. She has boxes of chocolates and biscuits hidden all over her house and eats mainly processed food. Her emotional state is one of anxiety and she comfort eats on a regular basis.
- Cause: in regression work she revealed that, when she was a child, her mother told her that she must finish the food on her plate. Her mother also told her that there would come a time when there would be no more food.
- Explanation: she accepted this at a subconscious level to be literally true and ate to prepare herself for that day when there was no more food.

HABITUAL EATING

- Subject: a 35-year-old man was terrified he was going to have a heart attack. He had a hiatus hernia in his chest so was having chest pain and he was also five stone overweight. He had witnessed his father having a heart attack. He seemed to be set in his thinking that he was going to go the same way and so ate comfort food habitually as if to prove himself right.
- Cause: at deeper levels this man was very angry at his father's death. He felt angry with himself and the fact that he could not have helped him. He took on negative beliefs about himself – one of them being that going the same way was a form of self-punishment.

Explanation: this man was clearly developing behaviours to prove himself right. His eating became more and more habitual as he constantly needed to comfort himself. It seemed that the angrier he became, the more he would eat to stuff the emotions down.

EATING FOR REASSURANCE

Subject: this 29-year-old woman was the product of a mixed-race marriage. She had an Asian father who was extremely authoritarian and an English mother. The marriage broke up because of differing cultural beliefs.

Cause: this woman's father felt that his daughter had nothing to offer. She never felt encouraged by him and also felt that she was to blame for her parents' split.

Explanation: she ate excessively for comfort and to reassure herself that she wasn't worthless. She worked extra hard to be accepted by society and of course by her father. Sadly her father was impossible to satisfy and it became a vicious circle.

EATING FOR ENGLAND

Subject: a 47-year-old man who worked hard during the day and when he went home at night could not stop eating.

Cause: this man was incredibly driven to be successful. He felt he was never good enough at school and was making up for it now. He was something of a perfectionist.

Explanation: his binge eating was a way of dealing with his loneliness and his inferiority complex. He coped by stuffing those feelings down with food when he was on his own in the evening and as a release mechanism after all his efforts at the office.

Are you an emotional eater? Are you someone who feels burdened by the past and eats for comfort to compensate? Are you easily touched by outside events that send you running to the biscuit bin? Do any of the following statements apply to you?

- 'I eat excessively when I am on my own.'
- 'I have no control over the way that I eat.'
- 'I eat more when I am happy.'
- 'I eat more when I am unhappy.'
- 'I think about food all the time.'
- 'I am not really honest with myself about my eating habits.'
- 'I always feel guilty after eating.'
- 'Food seems to rule my life.'
- 'I simply enjoy food so much I never feel full – I can't seem to stop.'
- 'I eat out of boredom.'
- 'Even when I lose weight I feel insecure. So what's the point?'
- 'My eating goes up and down with my emotions.'
- 'I eat when other people upset me.'
- 'It doesn't matter if I've lost weight – I never feel good about myself.'
- 'My mood is affected by what I eat.'
- 'I eat more in the winter than in the summer.'
- 'I eat huge amounts of food then feel guilty and starve myself for long periods.'
- 'I am ashamed of the way that I eat.'
- 'I avoid social gatherings because I wouldn't be able to stop eating.'
- 'I eat when I am in stressful situations.'

Are you an emotional eater?

Clearly the more of these you tick the greater the influence of your emotions on your eating. If you feel that your eating patterns are out of control and have taken over your life, I would suggest that you seek help as soon as possible to redress the balance and regulate them – there is so much that you can do to help yourself.

If you suffer from any of the following extreme eating patterns I would strongly suggest that you get help from a professional.

- 'I use diet pills or laxatives to control my weight.'
- 'I starve myself.'
- 'I don't feel I deserve to eat.'
- 'I exercise excessively to lose weight.'
- 'After binge eating I make myself vomit.'
- 'I feel much more in control when I don't eat.'
- 'I have an intense fear of gaining weight.'
- 'I am completely secretive about what I eat or don't eat.'
- 'I eat vast amounts of food and I am totally unable to stop myself.'
- 'I think I have an eating disorder.'

Over the next month monitor your emotional experience with food. Jot down on a daily basis how you feel. You may want to explore where some of your feelings and behaviours have come from. So take a trip down memory lane to find out. Write it all down in your journal. Watch out for any emotional states that are more familiar than others – for example, anxiety or anger. Are there certain times of the month when you feel particularly emotional? You may want to be particularly on the look out for emotional triggers.

Angry

Happy

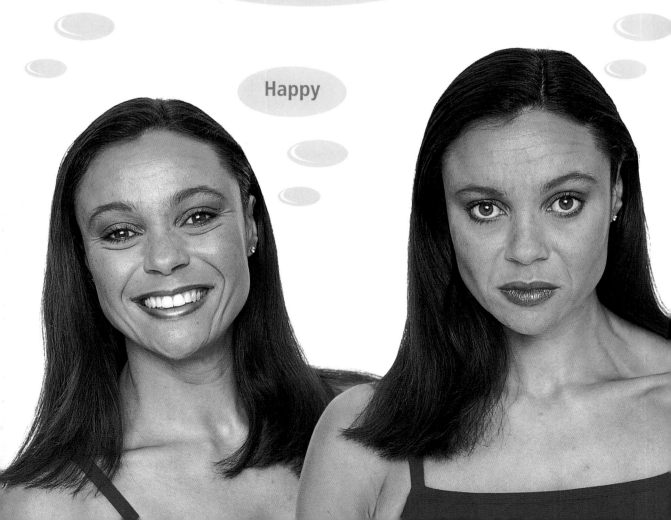

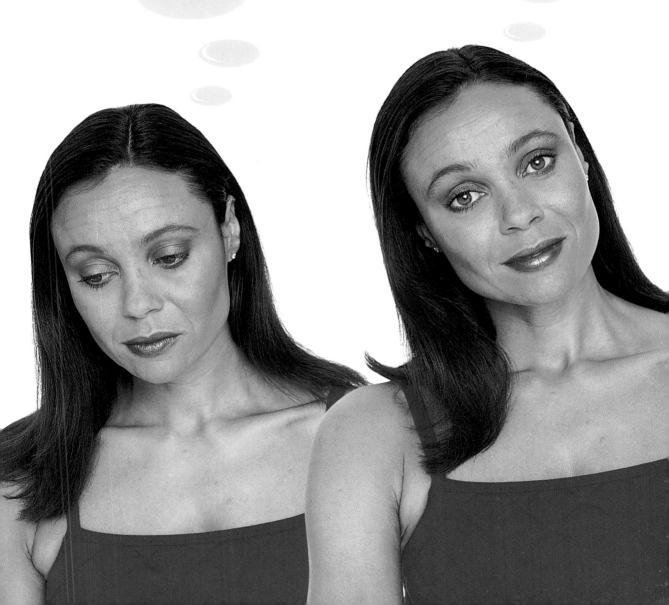

Emotional Triggers

Everything we do in life is a result of something that happens in the mind at a neurological level. We take in information through our senses, and that information sometimes forms triggers. A trigger is an internal reaction to an external stimulus. It works a bit like a light switch, with the stimulus switching on a specific neurological response. Triggers are very much linked to memories; they can be positive or negative and they can produce extreme states of mind such as phobic reactions. The sensory stimulus that consistently triggers a state is called an anchor. It may be something you see (visual), hear (auditory), feel (kinaesthetic), taste (gustatory), or smell (olfactory) that triggers an internal state or perhaps a memory of some kind.

Anchors

The sight of roses reminds me of my anniversary. Diana Ross's music brings on feelings of nostalgia. Going to my son's school brings back smells, sights and sounds that I recognize from my own childhood. The smell of coffee makes my mouth water. A traffic light on red means stop.

Roses, Diana Ross, coffee, these are just some of my anchors; and I've shown you what it is that they trigger. (I'd added the red traffic light to show that some anchors are shared by all of us.) Now, what about food triggers.

The smell of Caribbean food reminds me of my West Indian origins and the comfort of home (incidentally, the sight of boiled gammon and cabbage also reminds me of home – that's my Irish side). A bar of Turkish Delight chocolate reminds me of Friday evenings as a kid when all my family would be together – my father brought us home a treat every Friday. As for rhubarb – yuck. It reminds me of my parents' back garden.

They grew it there and we had it for pudding most days (it seemed). I can still taste how stringy it was. And if I ever hear the phrase 'eat your vegetables' I always remember that I would do exactly the opposite when I was a child; I didn't like the taste of them and didn't care that they were good for me.

Anchors are established over a lifetime and often we are completely unaware that we are reacting to them or of the degree to which they affect our lives. They are essentially a form of 'stimulus response conditioning' and they have a tremendous impact on our thinking and our behaviour from moment to moment as well as being directly linked to habitual behaviour. Anchors have a profound effect on your eating behaviour. Clearly the sight of a chocolate bar is a red rag to a chocoholic. A large plate of food equally so to the overeater who has been taught to eat everything even when they're not hungry. Put a plate of sugary treats in front of someone with a sweet tooth and you are asking for trouble.

Food Anchors

Think about your experience with food. What sights, sounds, tastes, smells, feelings can trigger emotional states that enable you to control your eating patterns in a positive way? When are you triggered to eat for reasons other than hunger? What sensory experiences create states of mind that result in negative eating patterns? Make a list of your food triggers.

Make a decision to become even more aware of any anchors that trigger off negative states of mind that affect your eating behaviour. For example, every morning I put the alarm clock on snooze so that I can sleep in until the last moment. And then I really have to hurry, which triggers an anxious state of mind as I fly out of the house without any breakfast. The result is that by mid-morning my blood-sugar level is low and so when the tea trolley comes round, I'm starving and I fill up on biscuits and buns.

How could you change this situation around and make the alarm clock an anchor for healthy eating?

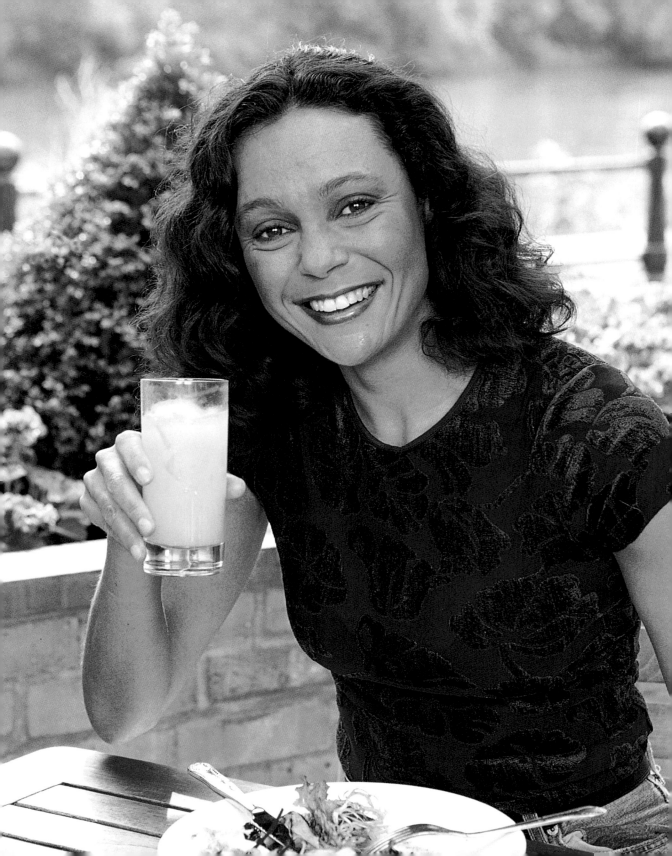

Food Anchors, Environmental Anchors

Think about the environmental anchors you have created for yourself; the home, for example, the office or the gym. Do you find home a relaxing place when you come in from a day's work or is it just as stressful? What are the food triggers here? Does a nice glass of wine relax you when you get through the front door, or is it straight to the biscuit barrel for a bit of comfort. What about the office? Is your environment such that you are driven to the chocolate-vending machine by the trigger of a stressful phone call or to alleviate the boredom you feel, or to appease your anxiety at having to meet a deadline?

Monitor your experience for a week in your various environments and become aware of their respective triggers and your responses to them. Start to think about ways to bring about change at home and at work. For

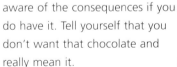

Create your own anchors for life.

example, if you are a chocoholic and home is where you binge, then ban chocolate from the house. The same goes for alcohol. Find other activities to distract you – something else that you enjoy and can focus on. If you find that you feel deprived keep reminding yourself of the long-term benefits of not eating chocolate. Be aware of the consequences if you do have it. Tell yourself that you don't want that chocolate and really mean it.

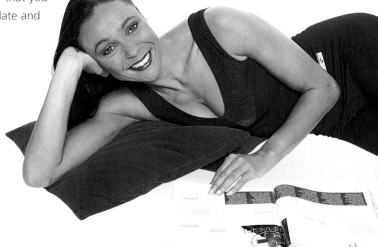

In order to change your relationship with food you need to be aware of your emotional triggers. And you need to realize that you can create your own anchors if you want to. You can do this by training yourself to focus on more positive states of mind.

You can create and build up your own anchors for more controlled eating patterns and you can choose the states you would rather have instead of the states that haven't served you well in the past. When you start building up your own anchors you are imprinting good feelings on your computer-like mind and training it to go in a new direction. It is important as you stack up anchors to be patient – as with anything you try to learn in life it takes time to fully assimilate them.

You might have noticed that in a number of exercises I told you to squeeze your non-dominant hand in order to 'lock in' an experience. What you are doing is setting up an association of the positive state with the sensation of squeezing your hand. You could also use visual symbols or a powerful word or phrase.

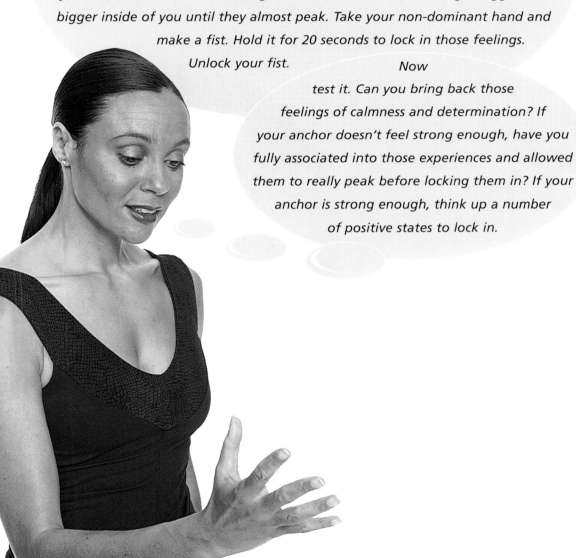

*Make
a list of states that would help you manage and
control your weight – for example, it would help to be calm,
relaxed, determined, controlled, focused – take each state at a time and
recall a time when you experienced it. Relive each experience as if you were
back there now. See what you saw, hear what you heard and feel what you felt. As
you become aware of the feelings focus on them and let them get bigger and
bigger inside of you until they almost peak. Take your non-dominant hand and
make a fist. Hold it for 20 seconds to lock in those feelings.
Unlock your fist.*

*Now
test it. Can you bring back those
feelings of calmness and determination? If
your anchor doesn't feel strong enough, have you
fully associated into those experiences and allowed
them to really peak before locking them in? If your
anchor is strong enough, think up a number
of positive states to lock in.*

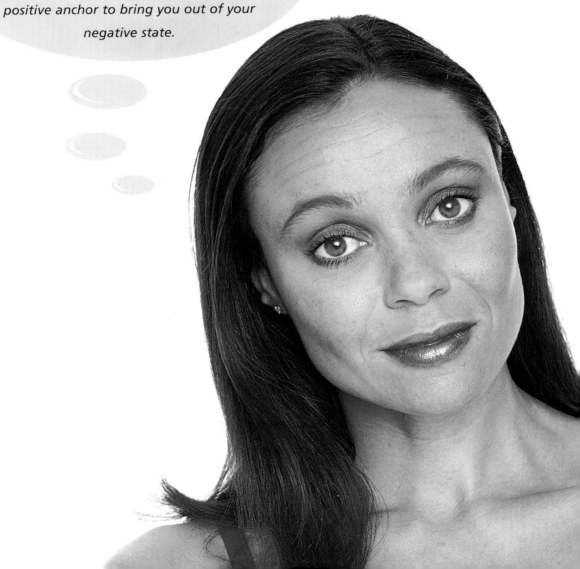

Think of your eating experiences. Make a list of states that have not been useful to you or that trigger negative behaviour.

Create a positive anchor that would be really useful to get you out of this negative frame of mind. Recall the positive experience; relive it and lock it in. Think of a negative state but don't anchor it. Relive it, and as you find yourself in this state fire off your positive anchor to bring you out of your negative state.

Sit in a comfortable position and count yourself down to relaxation. Every time you count a number, take your attention to all your body parts; keep telling yourself to slow down and relax.

Think of a challenging situation in the future. As you focus on this situation be aware of how you feel as this event looms. What happens to your eating as a result of those feelings? Do you eat more or less? Now bring your attention to how you might have felt and behaved in the past. Ask yourself if you still want to feel or behave this way.

You can intervene by using your imagination to focus on what you would rather feel and do instead. See yourself as you wish to be. Hear what you would hear; feel what you would feel. Make the picture as compelling as possible. Make the colours brighter, the picture clearer; bring it closer to you or take it farther away from you – whichever you find most comfortable. Imagine now that you are stepping into the picture and fully experience those feelings. Allow them to get bigger and bigger until they almost peak. Step out of the picture but bring the feelings with you. Turn now and look at the picture. Then take your non-dominant hand and lock those feelings into your body and see the picture at the same time.

Practise this exercise every day.

Beliefs affect your emotions and
therefore how you feel about yourself.

What Do You Believe?

Beliefs are ideas that you hold to be true – whether they are true or not.
Our beliefs can change and develop throughout our lifetime; but we also
have core beliefs. Most often these core beliefs will have developed from
when we were very young. Certainly most of the decisions you have made
about food will have been based on your childhood experiences, unless
you have changed those beliefs over time. Here are some real-life
examples:

- 'I believe that I will always be fat.'
- 'I must always eat what is in front of me.'
- 'I must never waste food.'
- 'I will never have a good relationship with food.'
- 'Food is the only thing that will comfort me when I am
  feeling down.'

Beliefs affect your emotions and therefore how you feel about
yourself; they can empower you or limit you in life. However, you can
change your limiting beliefs if you wish. You do this by doubting their
validity and by focusing on what you would rather believe instead.

Habitual Behaviour

Every experience you have leaves an imprint on your cortex, which is the
brain's 'receiving station' for information. Every time you repeat an
experience the imprint becomes stronger – it is very much like a path
being worn in your mind. The more you repeat a thought or a behaviour
the easier it becomes, until soon you can do it unconsciously. And at this
point it has become a habit.

Write a list of your current beliefs about food. Tick those that empower you and mark a cross next to those that limit you. Now choose one of each and write them down. Ask yourself this question, 'Is this belief really true?' Explore your experience with these beliefs. Where did you learn them? What lets you know whether they are true or not true? If you continue to hold on to these beliefs what will be the result? If it is not what you want, what would you rather believe instead? For example, 'I would rather believe that I am in full control of my eating habits', or 'I would rather believe that I can successfully lose weight.'

Imagine living out that new belief. For example, see and feel yourself in complete control of your eating. See what you would see (a trimmer, fitter you?). Hear what you would hear (praise – from yourself and other people?). Feel what you would feel (happier, more confident?).

All habitual behaviour is learned behaviour. Think about the things that you do automatically. You had to learn how to walk, talk and brush your teeth at some point. Think of young children doing those things; think of them in the middle of learning how. If you are a car driver or the owner of a bicycle you will know that you had to go through the learning process before you could drive or ride automatically. It is the same with eating patterns. The way you eat today is the result of how you learned to eat in the past. You certainly did not come into the world eating compulsively or gulping your food down or comfort eating; you have developed eating behaviours and then repeated them until they became automatic. Habitual behaviour can be a thought or an external behaviour (a movement or action). A habit might have its origins in a belief that you hold, which could be

Behaviours become habitual through repetition.

empowering or limiting, or it may be a response to your emotions – for example, every time you're unhappy or stressed you eat a chocolate bar because you believe it will make you feel better. Indeed habits work even more powerfully when emotions are involved. This is because we have a need to make ourselves feel better in some way; the brain finds a way to feel pleasure. Emotional eating develops into habitual behaviour because every time the stress response is triggered, you feel bad about yourself or in need of comfort you head for pleasurable states, normally in the biscuit tin. Most habits have their roots in our early years; but we build on and reinforce those early roots so that in time habitual behaviours and thought processes become unconscious.

The habitual behaviour you have today is a response to what you learned yesterday.

What Are Your Current Eating Habits?

- 'I eat when I'm not hungry.'
- 'I eat until I feel like I'm going to burst.'
- 'I'm always calorie counting.'
- 'I'm always on a diet.'
- 'I worry about food all the time.'
- 'I eat in front of the computer.'
- 'I eat in front of the telly in the evening.'
- 'I eat when I am on the run.'
- 'I always avoid eating fruit and vegetables.'
- 'I never have time for breakfast.'
- 'I get on the scales every morning.'
- 'I gulp my food down.'
- 'I never feel satisfied.'

If you always do what you have always done you will always get what you have always got.

They say that old habits die hard but if you choose to you can unlearn your habitual behaviour, creating new pathways in your mind and establishing positive behaviour patterns instead. Some people think they will never change, and of course the result is they remain stuck in their old ways. The longer you continue with old patterns the more set they become and the more difficult it is to change them.

So if you want to make a change in your life you need to do something different. Pick one of the statements that you ticked and answer the following questions.

- How much do you want to change your habit – a little, a lot, or can you live with it? Find out how motivated you are.
- Is this habit good for you? Explore what the habit actually does for you, what you see, hear and feel as a result of it.
- Where did you learn this habit? Explore the experiences that caused you to develop it.
- What purpose does this habit serve for you? Discover its underlying motivation: perhaps it creates a feeling of comfort or security.
- What will be the result if you continue with this habit? Think about the future and the consequences of your habitual behaviour. Again, imagine what you will see, hear and feel as a result.
- What new habit would you rather have instead?

Now write your findings in your journal.

If you want to change your habits you need to be patient. The time it takes will depend on how open you are to change, how much you want to change and how long you take to put new skills into place. Sometimes when we try to learn new things old habits get in the way. It seems impossible to fight the temptations of yesterday but it is essential not to be hard on yourself if you do succumb. Simply acknowledge what has happened, look at the reasons for the lapse and think about the long-term consequences if you revert to your old habits; then get yourself back on track and establish the new habits that you would rather have instead. When you do this you are training your mind to develop and reinforce new thought patterns.

The first step to changing a habit is to be aware of it and to learn the patterns that cause you to perpetuate it such as where, when and why you do it. The next step is to make a committed decision to find ways and means to change it so that you can develop a more positive eating pattern and reinforce your commitment to making those changes. Only when you are aware of what you are doing, can you change it, because only then do you get the chance to think twice before repeating your old behaviour.

Think Twice

- Think twice when you do your weekly shop. If you don't think, you are likely to wander up and down the aisle of your favourite supermarket throwing anything you fancy into your trolley. Write a list beforehand and make sure you stick to it.

- Think twice before putting any unnecessary food into your trolley. I know that two packets of biscuits for the price of one is an enticing bargain, but do you really need that extra packet? Just imagine what that extra packet will look like on your body. If you are a binge eater you need to think twice before you put any foods that you binge on into your trolley. My motto is a simple one: if you want to be trim don't eat the foods that make you fat – cut them out. That may seem a little harsh but feeling and being overweight is harsher.

- Think twice about the quality of the food that you habitually eat. Look out for added sugar, fats and salt; look at your ratio of fresh food to processed food. Make the decision to eat fresh, healthy foods. Be aware of the range of foods you eat – do you always eat the same things? Explore different food options and always ask yourself, 'Is this good for my body?' If the answer is 'no', then don't put the food in your basket.

- Think twice about the treats that you give yourself. If you can minimize the amount of biscuits and chocolate you eat then great, but most people don't find it easy. Find other ways to treat yourself instead. It may feel like deprivation when you cannot have treats, but I maintain that real deprivation means feeling fat, miserable and guilty because you have indulged – rather than feeling happy and proud of your accomplishments.

- Think twice about what you eat when you are out and about. Instead of stopping for calorie-laden fried chicken or a hamburger go for healthier alternatives: wholemeal sandwiches, salads or maybe try a noodle bar...

- Think twice before you eat. Ask yourself, 'Am I really hungry? How do I know that I am hungry?' Measure your hunger on the dial that you imagined in the earlier exercise. And if you are not hungry, explore your emotional state – is it urging you to eat? Break the pattern by doing something else instead: visualize your dreams, play some music, go for a walk, do a crossword, get creative.
- Think twice before eating when you feel low, and realize that you can get yourself out of this state by firing off your positive anchors. Or do something to change your state. If you need to get something off your chest, talk to a friend or write your feelings down in a letter. (Don't send it though – just use it as a therapeutic tool to express your emotions.)
- Think twice about the way you eat. Are you shovelling it in too quickly? Or are you simply eating too much? Make the decision to eat slowly and only until you are comfortable. If you don't know if you are comfortable, stop eating and wait a while; and if you don't feel hungry again don't eat any more.
- Think twice before jumping on the scales. They form negative associations with your self-image. Think of all the negative suggestions and reinforcements you give yourself when the scales are a few pounds over. Find other ways to measure your success: be aware of how you feel; take measurements of your waist, hip, thighs, bust instead; see how your clothes fit you.

The following 'habit-buster' – 'the swish pattern' – is very popular with neuro-linguistic practitioners. It encourages the brain to work in a new direction. It takes around 21 days of practice to create a new habit. Go for it!

Think of a habit that you would like to change. Imagine that you are in a cinema with a good view of the screen. The screen is blank. In a moment it will flicker with an image of you just about to do what you want to stop doing – for example, just about to reach for the biscuit tin. Imagine stepping into the scene to get an idea of what you are feeling. Step out of the picture.

Now create an image of what you would rather be doing instead. Get a sense of the pleasure that you feel by doing something positive. Try it for size. Adjust the visual intensity. Step out of the picture. Shrink this picture and place it in the top right-hand corner of the screen.

The objective is to replace the original picture with the new positive picture. The cue word is 'swish', and when you say it you superimpose the new picture on the old one and the new picture shrinks. Make the new picture explode with colour. Blank the screen. And now say 'swish' ten times, blanking the screen between each swish.

Try to bring the original picture back. If the swish is effective the old picture will not come back. If it does, see how you can make the new picture even more compelling – make it brighter and clearer, put a big smile on your face and swish again until the old picture does not try to come back. Now step into the new picture and try it on for size. If it feels good let the feelings get bigger and when they feel like they are going to peak, step out of the picture and bring the positive feelings with you as you now turn to look at that picture. Take your non-dominant hand and make a fist and lock those feelings in along with the pictures in your mind.

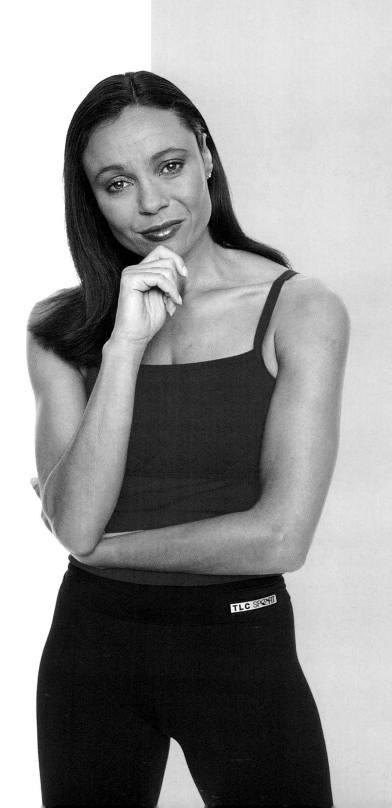

Chapter 5

The Food You Eat

Your body is made up of trillions of cells that are constantly regenerating. Cells mass together to create tissue in your body, forming organs, nerves, muscles and bones. We also have a number of fat cells in our body, dictated initially by genetics but increasing in number and size throughout life as our lifestyle exerts its influence. Each fat cell contains hormones, nutrients, and oxygen, all ready to be metabolized to produce energy. We store fat under our skin, in the muscles and around our internal organs. The body has the capacity to accumulate almost endless amounts of fat. When we gain weight our fat cells fill up; when weight is lost they release fat and reduce in size.

The cells in your body are very much influenced by what you eat; give them good nourishment and they will function optimally for you.

The Food You Eat

But how do we know what optimum nourishment is? If you have been a follower of diet culture over the years there is no doubt that you have picked up a lot of information about nutrition; you are probably something of an expert. You will have realized by now that no single diet works for everyone. This tells us that we all have metabolic differences; we process food differently. 'One man's meat is another man's poison' – when it comes to diet there is no truer expression. The aim for each individual is to discover what works for them; what provides optimum nourishment for their body. The result: metabolic balance, a healthy amount of fat in the fat cells and, ultimately, your ideal bodyweight.

> Every individual processes food differently.

This chapter offers some basic nutritional advice. There is no advice on calorie restriction because, as I have said, I believe that no single diet works for everyone. If you have followed the previous chapters you will now be exercising control over your eating behaviour, you will be aware of how you eat and of any psychological attachments you have to food. You will now be training yourself to think before you eat and you will now be more in tune and connected with your body's needs. Your new awareness has opened up the possibility of change.

Your Food Diary

Now is the time to start a food diary and make a record of what you eat; and pay attention to the quality as well as the quantity – because often we lie to ourselves about both. Once you have put it all down on paper – honestly – you can evaluate what you need to do and make changes where they are needed.

The Basic Rules for Weight Loss

The rules for weight loss are pretty basic. If you are inactive and you eat too much or eat for reasons other than hunger, the food that you are eating is excess – you will wear it on your body. If you are a veteran dieter you might have undermined your normal appetite and hunger signals to achieve your weight-loss goals. This might have led to a degree of restraint in the short term but you wouldn't have been able to keep it up in the long term. But keep focusing on eating only when you are physically hungry and stopping when you are comfortably full and you will begin the process of retraining your body to move towards its natural bodyweight.

So, my first piece of advice: eat only what your body needs. My own strategy is to eat three meals a day and – only if I need them – two healthy snacks. If I'm not hungry I don't have the snacks. I believe that this is all my body needs to function optimally at a healthy bodyweight. First thing in the morning I eat a piece of spelt bread with Marmite on it and an apple; mid-morning I have a bigger breakfast, which could be ham and eggs or an omelette and salad. I eat a late lunch at about two o'clock: it could be soup and a rice salad or some other sort of salad that contains both protein and carbohydrate, or I dive for the nearest noodle bar. I have a snack around five o'clock if I am hungry. This is normally raw vegetables and a dip. At about eight o'clock in the evening I have a supper of fish or chicken and lots of vegetables. I have a glass of wine every evening, I drink a cup of boiled water with a lemon segment to start the day and I drink lots of camomile or peppermint tea all day.

Eat only what your body needs.

I like to have a fairly substantial meal early in the day because it gives me a sense of fullness that I carry around with me throughout the day. I don't feel the need to snack as a result. I leave food on the plate if I am feeling full and no one can persuade me to eat what I don't need. (Not even my mum.) This strategy may not work for everyone so you need to work out what works for you.

Don't eat the foods that make you fat.

My second piece of advice is: don't eat the foods that make you fat – eat the right foods for your body. I can hear you saying 'Hmm, that's a bit obvious.' But how many of you eat the very foods that make you fat because of food cravings, bad habits or not knowing about the hidden fats in foods? Now, if you were to go to the doctor with the symptoms of a 'proper' illness such as diabetes or even heart disease you would be told to avoid certain foods. Well, if the symptom of your 'illness' is excess fat on your body, why not treat being overweight in the same way. If you have food cravings that are causing you to eat uncontrollably, and this is having a detrimental effect on your body, then cut out those foods.

But you may say, 'I feel deprived.' Firstly, you need to think about which is most important – the long-term goal, which is a slimmer you, or a few minutes' gratification stolen by stuffing your face (and feeling dreadful afterwards)? Tucking into foods that are not doing your body any good is the cause of real deprivation; feeling fat and miserable is real deprivation. I would strongly recommend that you remind yourself of your goal and do something to take your mind off the food that you crave. The cravings will soon pass. Secondly, those cravings need to be addressed at a physiological level. Once you have achieved metabolic balance you are likely to lose those cravings. In the meantime you should focus on how you eat, what you eat and your long-term target of a slimmer you.

I've set out my basic strategies for weight loss, now let's look closely at what you will be eating. To begin with, food is made up of three major macronutrients (put simply, substances that you require in relatively large amounts): proteins, fats and carbohydrates.

Proteins

Present in every cell – your skin, nails, bones, blood and of course your muscles – protein is, after water, the most plentiful substance in your body. Described as the basic building block of the body, it plays a major role in the growth and repair of body tissues – in fact everything you are made up of. Protein also works to maintain an effective immune and hormonal system.

Amino Acids

Proteins are broken down by digestive enzymes and absorbed into the blood as amino acids to be used by the body. Amino acids link together to form a chain of structures giving each protein its specific characteristics, be it nail, muscle, or a hormone such as insulin. There are 23 amino acids and eight of them are essential. These eight essential amino acids need to be present in the food we eat for complete protein integration. Basically, the better the balance of amino acids, the better the use you make of that protein.

Good Protein Foods

Lean organic beef, lamb, rabbit, venison, ostrich, whey, chicken, turkey, eggs, bass, mackerel, sardines, trout, tuna, cod, tofu, soya products are all good protein foods. Avoid processed foods such as sausages, shop-bought hamburgers, bacon, pepperoni and corned beef.

Protein can also come in the form of shakes and powders. These are usually based on milk solids, soya or brewers' yeast. Diets based on these shakes and powders can be harmful: they are often too low in calories and devoid of essential fatty acids. You may lose weight in the short term but you are likely to have lost lean muscle tissue and develop deficiencies in the long term.

Chemical Messengers

Essential amino acids are also instrumental in the formation of neurotransmitters, which are the body's chemical messengers. They work like couriers, delivering messages to different parts of the body. Neurotransmitters determine how you feel and have a powerful affect on your mood. There are hundreds of chemical messengers in the body but among the best known are:

- ADRENALINE is the fight-or-flight hormone that motivates you to act in response to stress.
- SEROTONIN is responsible for mood – lack of it can make you feel blue. You can produce serotonin from the amino acid tryptophan, which is found in foods such as turkey, fish, avocados and bananas.
- ACETYLCHOLINE is a neurotransmitter responsible for improving the mental faculties.
- NORADRENALINE and DOPAMINE are the neurotransmitters that make you feel in control.
- GABA (from 'gamma-aminobutyric acid') is a relaxant neurotransmitter.

Protein also encourages the production of a hormone called glucagon, which balances excess insulin. It also stimulates the liver to release glucose, which has been stored as glycogen – in other words it promotes using stored fat as energy. Glucagon and the hormone insulin work together in a see-saw action to maintain blood glucose at a required level: glucagon increases it; insulin decreases it.

Optimum Protein Nutrition

Your diet must include all the essential amino acids for optimum nutrition. But not all protein foods contain all the essential amino acids; these are called 'incomplete proteins' and they are lentils, beans, pulses, nuts and seeds. However, eat them in combination with other foods such as grains, rice and soya and you will satisfy your body's requirements and eat a

*Make
a note of all protein foods that you
eat on daily basis. Are you getting enough
protein foods in your diet? Are they complete
proteins? Are the protein foods that you
eat fresh or organic?*

complete protein meal. You don't have to eat them in the same meal as previously thought, but in the same day.

As far as quantity is concerned, if you eat too much protein it is stored as fat. You need to eat around one gram of protein per kilogram of bodyweight or, alternatively, a palmful of protein – as much protein as it takes to cover the palm of your hand to the same depth as your palm. Switch off the hunger signals with a protein snack to fill the gap: how about tinned mackerel and sardines or a hard-boiled egg. Or combine protein with a carbohydrate and essential fat: raw vegetables with a tahini dip or turkey slices with vegetable sticks.

Here are some more protein suggestions:

- Go for protein foods that are fresh or organic. Lean, organic, grass-fed meats and organic poultry are more nutrient-dense, which means you feel the need to eat less.
- Oily fish – sardines, salmon, mullet and mackerel – contain the essential fatty acids omegas 3 and 6, which are believed to improve conditions such as heart disease and promote feelings of satiety.
- Vegetarians can choose from soya-based products, (low-fat) cheeses, eggs, tofu, nuts, seeds, pulses and beans. Eat beans together with a grain for a complete protein meal, or try: pasta with chickpeas, almond nut butter on wholemeal spelt bread, brown rice and lentils, stir-fried tofu with rice, stir-fried vegetables with walnuts, almond slivers on brown rice or vegetables and Soya products such as tofu.

Fats

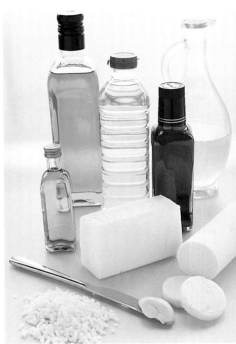

Have you ever sat down to a low-fat meal, eaten loads and still felt hungry afterwards – so you find something else to eat to fill the gap! In which case you might not have been eating the essential fats your body needs to feel full. Over the last two decades we have been indoctrinated with the idea that fat is bad for us. Gurus have promoted their low-fat diets by promising that you will lose those extra pounds for ever. The theory is that fat – unlike carbohydrates and proteins – is calorie-dense (it is the most concentrated form of energy) and if we only eat minimal amounts we must lose weight. The thinking has changed because now we can see the results of 20 years of low-fat dieting: poor skin condition, cracked nails, lifeless hair, wind and bloating, poor digestion, constipation, depression, aching joints, obesity and insulin imbalance...to name just a few.

Fat is essential for the protection of our internal organs for the production of the hormones oestrogen and progesterone and for carrying those hormones around the body. It is also a carrier of fat-soluble vitamins such as A and E as well as D and K. And fat, as was mentioned above, is a vital energy source. It is also thought that fat is a useful resource for weight management: the right amount of body fat works to decrease the appetite, so you don't feel hungry.

Next we are going to see that it is the type of fat you eat that makes all the difference to good health and an ideal bodyweight.

Two Different Types of Fat

Fat is divided into two groups: saturated and unsaturated. Saturated fats come from animal-derived sources such as meat, butter, cream and dripping; they are more concentrated and are solid at room temperature. Unsaturated fats are divided into two groups: monounsaturated and polyunsaturated. Unsaturated fats come mainly from plants and fish oils. Plant-derived sources are olive oil, vegetable oils (such as flaxseed, sunflower, safflower and rapeseed oils) and nut oils. Fish sources come from the more oily fish: mackerel, sardine, tuna. Unsaturated fats are liquid at room temperature.

Fatty Acids

When you eat fat, your digestion breaks it down into glycerol and fatty acids. Amongst the many functions of these essential fatty acids is that they help the body to resist illness by supporting the immune system. They also support the reproductive and central nervous systems.

Fatty acids have a molecular structure that consists of a chain of carbon atoms. Each carbon atom has a single linking 'arm' with another carbon atom, plus it has one or more free 'arms'. When all the free 'arms' are attached to hydrogen atoms, then the fat becomes saturated with hydrogen and is called a saturated fat.

However, if the free arms on the carbon atoms are only attached to other carbon atoms (or double bonded), they cannot be saturated with hydrogen and are therefore unsaturated fats. Fatty acids with only one double bond are monosaturated; those with two or more double bonds are polyunsaturated. Even so, the double bonded molecules in unsaturated fats can still take up hydrogen and so can be artificially saturated with hydrogen – this process is called hydrogenation. When this happens an unsaturated fat becomes a hydrogenated fat.

The problem is that the more saturated a fat becomes, the harder the body finds it to metabolize and the more likely it is to be stored in your fat cells. Some common products that contain saturated fats are biscuits, cereal bars, spreads (especially low-fat ones) pastries and packaged foods.

There are concerns over hydrogenated fat, the production of which involves changing a liquid into a semi-solid fat by basically, and as the name suggests, adding hydrogen. For example, hydrogenated fat has be found to contribute to a number of disorders such as low birth weights,

Have you been on a low-fat diet? How did you find it? What kinds of fats are you putting in your body now? Go through your cupboards and fridge and check the fat content of the foods there. Are you getting enough of the vital omega 3 and omega 6 fatty acids in your diet? Do you feel full and satisfied after a meal or do you need to keep eating? What is your thinking now about fat?

decreased testosterone in men, heart disease and cancer. Some margarines and other hydrogenated vegetable oils interfere with cholestorol levels and the metabolism of essential fatty acids.

What kinds of fat should we eat? It's okay to eat a small amount of saturated fat (butter, cream) but you should avoid hydrogenated fats completely. (Note that you will find hidden hydrogenated fats in pies, pasties, pastries, cakes, biscuits, breaded foods such as fish fingers and chicken nuggets, sauces, salad oils, cereals, bread, margarines and more.) The fats that you really need to include in your diet are the unsaturated fats, and preferably the polyunsaturated ones.

Polyunsaturated fats are better because they contain the two essential fatty acids omega 3 and omega 6, which are highly recommended on a regular basis. These fats should be incorporated in any weight-control programme because they work as natural appetite suppressants. They produce the hormone cholecystokinin (or CCK), in the stomach, which sends a signal to the brain to indicate satiety. They also increase fat metabolism so that more stored fat is burned as energy. Omega 3 is also known to increase sensitivity to insulin, the hormone that regulates blood sugar levels. Sources of polyunsaturates are oily fish such as mackerel, sardines, and also flaxseed oil, hempseed oil, nuts, seeds, grains and vegetables.

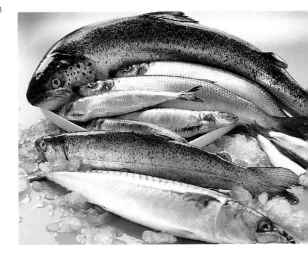

Here are some more suggestions:

- Go for foods that contain unsaturated fats.
- Go through your cupboards and throw out any foods that contain hydrogenated fats.
- Ensure that you include oily fish in your diet.
- If you are not getting the essential fatty acids in your diet, snack on flaxseeds or have a heaped tablespoonful of freshly ground seeds sprinkled on cereal; you can also try sesame, sunflower and pumpkin seeds. Alternatively, take a daily dessertspoon of flaxseed oil.
- Add oils that contain the essential omegas 3 and 6 to salad dressings; use red wine vinegar and white wine vinegar or lemon juice, garlic or coarse grain mustard. Instead of putting a knob of butter on your vegetables, drizzle flaxseed, walnut, hempseed or olive oil over them instead.
- Look after your oils by making sure the cap is tightly screwed on the bottle so that they aren't constantly exposed to oxygen. Store them in a cool, dark place such as the fridge. Buy them in glass bottles – dark glass is better than clear. Flaxseed oil must be refrigerated after opening and should only be purchased if it has been refrigerated.
- Use oils cold rather than hot: heating most oils makes them lose their nutritional value. Use olive oil for cooking.
- Buy lean organic meat or poultry whenever possible.
- Grill, bake or boil rather than frying.
- Eat fewer takeaways: fish and chips (sorry chaps), hamburgers and curries (if you must, go for a dry dish, such as lamb tikka or chicken tandoori with vegetables).

Carbohydrates

The other great dietary fallacy of the latter part of the last century concerns carbohydrate foods. Experts told us that the main macronutrient in our diet should be carbohydrate. Certainly a carbohydrate-rich diet has been proven vital for sports performance and other activities that require a high amount of energy. However, it has transpired that this type of diet does not suit most people, and it has resulted in an increase in disordered metabolisms, food intolerances and cravings. Increased carbohydrate consumption is also linked to the weight that we as a nation are putting on.

Carbohydrates are categorized as simple or complex. Simple carbohydrates include 'simple sugars' such as glucose, fructose, galectose, sucrose and lactose; these are abundant in table sugar, some fruit, honey and milk products. Pure white refined sugar provides energy but no other nutrients and mainly goes straight into the body's fat cells to be stored as energy; pure sugar is also found in sweet fizzy drinks.

Complex carbohydrates are made up of more complicated sugars, starches and fibre. They are a better fuel for the body, containing nutrients and fibre. When broken down to their finest form they are stored in the muscles and liver as glycogen that can be converted into energy.

Refined complex carbhohydrates are foods that have lost their rough coatings and fibres – they have had their husks and skins removed. They have been refined and, in the process, deprived of their vitamin and mineral content. As a result, they behave in the body like simple carbohydrates, and stimulate the production of insulin at the same rate. White flour (used to make white bread) and white rice, are examples of refined complex carbohydrate foods. Often these carbohydrates are combined with fats (especially hydrogenated fats) and white sugar to make them more tempting to the palate.

Simple and Refined-Complex Cabohydrates

Sugar, honey, white bread, white pasta, white rice, cakes, jams, biscuits, refined cereals with sugar coatings, sweet drinks, chocolate, alcohol, rice cakes, fruit and fruit juice.

Complex Carbohydrates

Wholegrains, brown rice, millet, rye, amaranth, quinoa, wholewheat pasta, corn, barley, brown bread, broccoli, spinach, chickpeas, lentils, turnips, aubergines, cauliflower, sweet potatoes, parsnips, squashes.

The difference between the two carbohydrates is that foods that contain simple sugars are very quickly absorbed into the blood stream and, in the process, stimulate a rapid release of the hormone insulin, whose job it is to keep blood sugar within its normal limits. With complex unrefined carbohydrates the release of sugar into the blood stream is more moderate and takes place over a longer period of time. When simple and refined complex carbohydrates are eaten, more insulin is excreted in order to regulate blood sugar levels. So the fundamental distinction of concern between simple and complex unrefined carbohydrates is that they raise blood sugar levels at different rates.

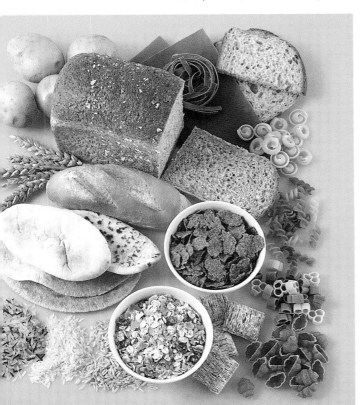

Different carbohydrates produce different responses in the body.

Fibre

Fibre is an essential part of a healthy eating programme, playing a crucial role in digestion. Fibre is found in complex carbohydrate foods such as grains, fruit, vegetables, seeds and nuts, with the greatest concentrations found in the skins and outer coatings of these foods. People who get plenty of fibre in their diets generally show a low incidence of bowel cancer, diabetes and obesity – fibre fills you up so you don't feel hungry. There are two types of fibre: soluble and insoluble. Soluble fibre dissolves easily in water and is broken down during digestion. It helps control the uptake of sugar by the blood and helps to push food through the digestive system. Psyllium husks are an excellent source of fibre.

The Glycaemic Index

The Glycaemic Index (GI) was originally devised to help diabetics to control their blood sugar level. The GI measures the degree to which a carbohydrate food will raise blood sugar and insulin levels (we have seen above that carbohydrates affect blood sugar levels at different rates). There are around 600 foods listed on the Glycaemic Index and each has a GI 'score'. The higher a food scores on the Glycaemic Index the more rapid is its release of sugar (and therefore insulin) into the blood stream. Normally the more refined a food is the higher its GI rating will be. Examples of refined foods are white rice, white bread, cereals, biscuits, cakes and sweets. But that is not always the case: some complex carbohydrate foods score very highly too. Although originally designed for diabetics, the GI is a great way for anyone to take control of their blood sugar level. It is important to emphasize that the GI concept should not be used alone, but alongside healthy eating guidelines.

(The list opposite shows just a few of the different kinds of foods on the Glycaemic Index, and I would highly recommend that you send away for the complete list. The address is given at the back of book, *see* p. 143.)

LOW GI	MODERATE GI	HIGH GI	VERY HIGH GI
Green vegetables	Whole rye bread	Pasta	Cornflakes
Fish	Barley	Oranges	Puffed rice
Seafood	Porridge	Peas	Rice cakes
Soya beans	Basmati rice	Baked beans	White bread
Meat and chicken	Buckwheat	Potatoes	Rice
Eggs	Pitta bread	Muesli	Shredded Wheat
Yoghurt	Apples	Ryvita	Parsnips
Milk	Kiwi	Popcorn	Sweetcorn
Cottage cheese	Beetroot		Bananas
Tahini	Kidney beans		Raisins
Seeds	Chickpeas		Apricots
Grapefruit	Skimmed milk		Mangoes
Plums	Low-fat yoghurt		Papaya
Peanuts			

Your energy, your sense of satiety, your mood, your body fat levels and your general health are greatly influenced by the type and the amount of sugar you consume. If you always eat foods that score high on the Glycaemic Index, or if you crave carbohydrate-rich foods, or if you have tried to lose weight on a low-fat, high-carbohydrate diet, you are probably suffering, or have suffered, from the over-production of insulin.

Insulin

The amount of insulin released by your body is related to what you eat. Insulin is a hormone secreted by the pancreas. It has a number of roles to play in the body. It has an effect on your appetite. It also plays a role in fat metabolism. But it plays its most vital role in the regulation and balancing of blood sugar (or glucose). The food you eat is broken down by digestive processes into blood sugar so it can be absorbed into the body. Insulin kicks in to regulate blood sugar and make use of it in the body. If you eat foods that are high in sugar, insulin has to be released faster and in higher quantities in order to regulate blood sugar levels. So if you consistently consume too much sugar, the digestive system is forced to secrete excess insulin to absorb it into the body.

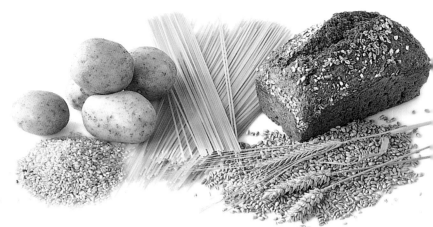

It is now recognized that it is not just excess fat in the diet that causes body fat levels to soar: carbohydrate also has a role to play. After insulin has done its job, any excess glucose in the body is shunted along to the fat cells for storage. Today, Western diets are high in both simple and complex carbohydrates but any excess of either can play havoc with this processing of sugars in the body. Eating too much carbohydrate-rich food – especially foods high on the Glycaemic Index – on its own without protein or fat can cause insulin production to jump rapidly as the body tries to keep blood sugar levels normal. Sometimes too much insulin is secreted, resulting in low blood sugar levels. This can affect your mood, and it can affect your appetite, bringing on feelings of hunger and cravings and thus the whole process starts all over again. When this cycle is repeated, the body's cells lose their sensitivity to insulin so that even more is needed to redress future imbalances, and in time this can lead to conditions such as hypoglycaemia, diabetes and obesity.

So both simple and complex sugars have an effect on insulin production and can lead to an overworked and therefore impaired pancreas. Simple sugars and foods high on the Glycaemic Index are the main culprits. Most of these types of foods carry little bulk and empty calories (calories that have little or no nutritional value), which can cause feelings of hunger. Complex carbohydrates that are rich in fibre and nutrients and are low on the Glycaemic Index cause a slower, more moderate rise in blood sugar levels – and they are what you should incorporate into your diet.

Carbohydrates and Mood

We looked earlier at the neurotransmitters that take messages from one nerve cell to another. Two of them, serotonin and noradrenaline, are 'mood-altering' chemicals. The body derives them from the foods that we eat, particularly from carbohydrates. As we have seen, certain carbohydrate

What is your experience of carbohydrate foods? Do you eat mostly simple or complex carbohydrates or a mixture of both? What is your ratio of carbohydrate to protein foods? What are the particular foods you feel the urge to eat? What times of day are you compelled to eat these foods? Do you always stick to the foods you know? How can you begin to change your carbohydrate intake?

foods can cause a sudden rise in blood sugar levels and it is this sudden fluctuation that produces a serotonin-high. But it only lasts for a short period of time before your insulin kicks in to regulate your blood sugar level. Your blood sugar level then drops causing seretonin levels to drop, making you feel 'down', which in turn makes you reach for the chocolates or coffee jar again. The best types of foods to balance serotonin levels are foods that score low to moderate on the Glycaemic Index. Serotonin is derived from the essential amino acid tryptophan which is found in high-protein foods such as turkey.

Here are some suggestions:

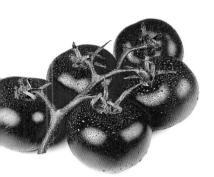

- Go for foods that rate low on the Glycaemic Index.
- Eat vegetables and grains.
- Choose foods that are natural and high in fibre: wholegrains and vegetables
- Avoid simple carbohydrates.
- Snack on low-GI fruits and vegetables.
- Combine carbohydrate foods with protein and essential fats.

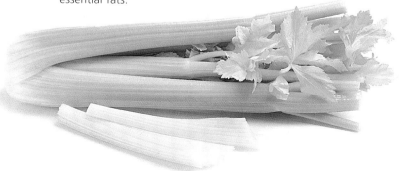

Fluids

You are 60 per cent water: two-thirds of your body and almost half your brain. Water provides the fluid that is vital for efficient functioning of the body both intracellularly (inside the cells) and extracellularly (blood plasma and saliva). Water is found in food especially fruit and vegetables, which are 90 per cent water. Drinking plenty of water will help you lose weight. It cleanses the body, ridding it of metabolic wastes and food residues, and it creates a sense of fullness if you drink it before a meal. Water has no calories but much is added to it. Sweetened drinks are heavily calorific, often having had pure sugar added to them. You can tell if you are drinking enough water by looking at the colour of your urine. It should be almost colourless except first thing in the morning. Drinking water is essential when you exercise because you lose fluids as you perspire, which can lead to dehydration.

Apart from pure water, the best sources of liquid are diluted juices and herbal and fruit teas. Keep alcohol and coffee to a minimum. Alcohol is carbohydrate-heavy and carries mainly empty calories, and coffee is a stimulant and diuretic, flushing water from the body. Keep a bottle of water with you all day.

Here are some guidelines:

- Drink eight to ten glasses of water a day – filtered or bottled.
- Drink herbal teas: camomile, valerian, Melissa (or lemon balm), peppermint, rose hip.
- Dilute shop-bought, pure fruit juices.
- Explore different drinks such as vegetable bouillon.
- Cut down on alcohol – no more than one or two glasses of wine per day.
- Green tea is said to aid weight loss by encouraging the body to burn fat. Don't drink too much though – it contains caffeine.

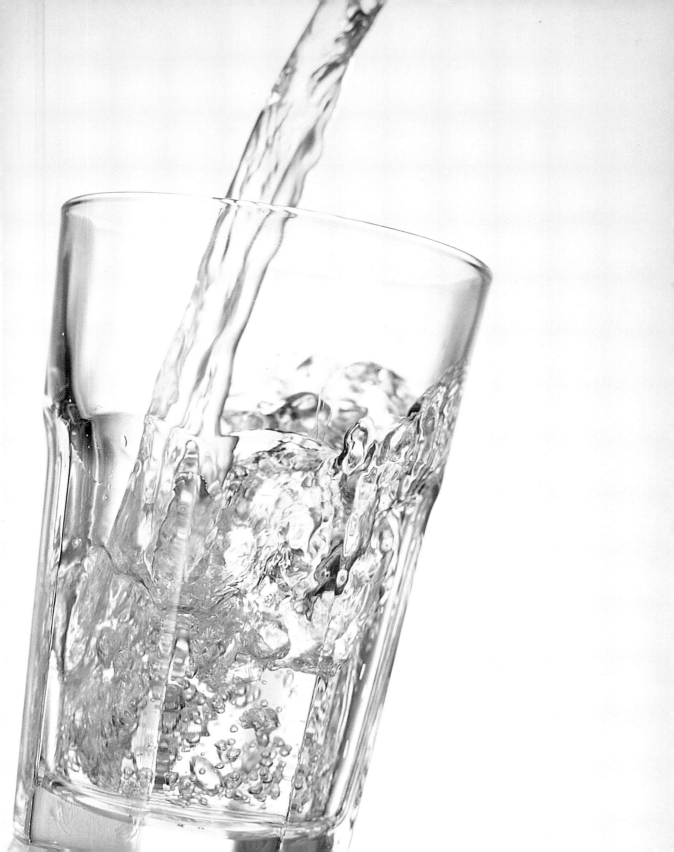

What Should We Eat?

Let me just repeat that I believe each individual has different metabolic needs, and that you need to discover what works for you. So, here is a summary of everything we have learned; it is especially pertinent if you have been on, or tempted by, a low-fat, high-carbohydrate diet.

You need to focus on eating an even balance of protein and carbohydrate foods and essential fats. Reduce carbohydrate intake to a modest amount and focus on getting most of it from vegetables and fruit with a low GI. Eat moderate amounts of grain. Choose foods that rate low on the Glycaemic Index – these will increase feelings of fullness. Slightly increase your protein intake and ensure you are eating a balanced amount of fish, meat and eggs. Eat complete proteins foods. Eat fish at least three times a week, particularly those that are rich in omegas 3 and 6: these will increase your cells' sensitivity to insulin and promote a feeling of satiety. Eat a palmful of top-quality protein with each meal.

For weight loss, ensure that you eat foods with a low GI score and plenty of fibre so you feel full. Combining carbohydrates and protein and modest amounts of the beneficial fats will promote feelings of fullness and slow the release of insulin into the body. If you are having a mid-morning or afternoon snack, go for combinations of protein, carbohydrates and fats. For example, raw vegetables and a healthy dip, walnuts, a piece of meat with vegetables. Eat only when you are hungry and stop eating when you are comfortably full. Avoid calorie counting: it is more important to eat the right amount of the right foods to control your hunger signals. If you do choose to restrict calories, don't reduce your intake by more than 15 per cent or your metabolism will slow down to preserve energy. It is also likely to reduce lean muscle mass through loss of lean muscle tissue and fluid – it is essential to maintain lean muscle mass. Eat the right kind of fats – especially in the form of extra virgin olive oil and walnut, safflower and flaxseed oils – and limit saturated fats. If you suffer from sugar cravings, ensure your diet is high in low-GI foods.

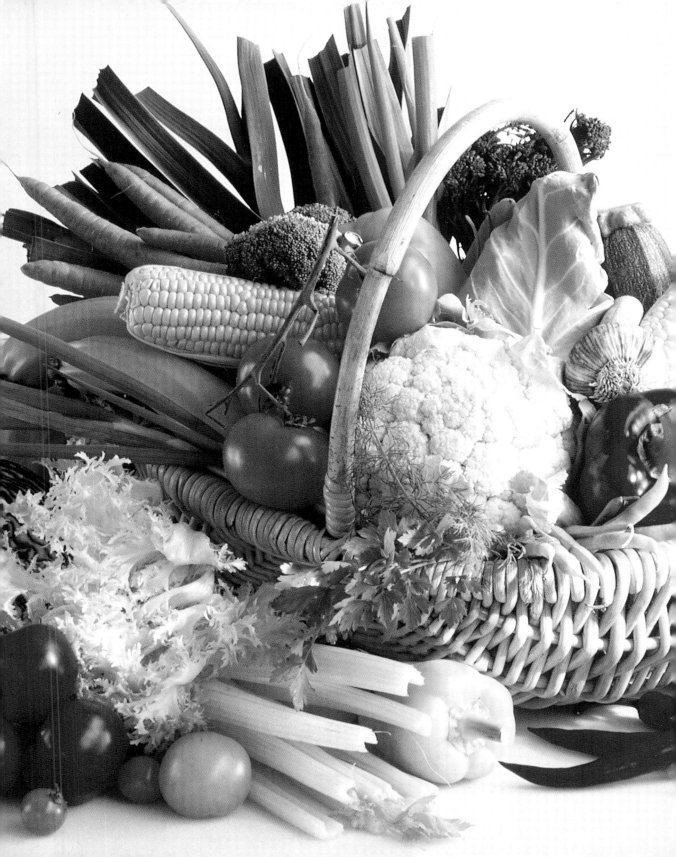

Finally, if you have any metabolic problems seek help from a good nutritional therapist or dietician. I personally advocate finding out about food intolerance through blood testing or blood typing or through an exploration of metabolic typing.

Once you have achieved your optimum weight and balanced your blood sugar level, focus on sticking to these nutritional guidelines, making modifications where necessary.

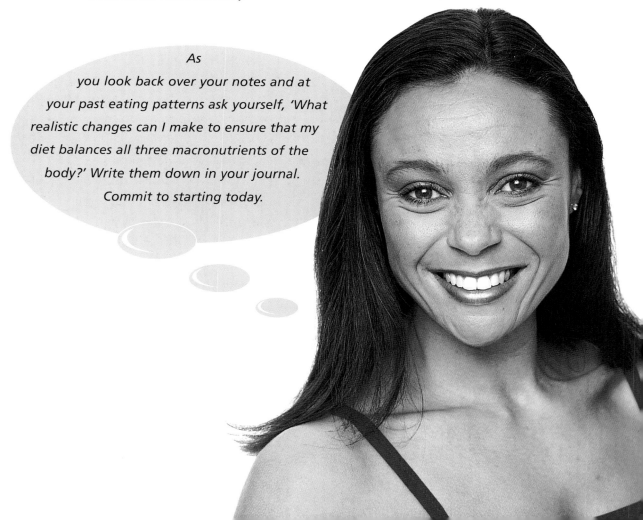

As you look back over your notes and at your past eating patterns ask yourself, 'What realistic changes can I make to ensure that my diet balances all three macronutrients of the body?' Write them down in your journal. Commit to starting today.

Herbs and Weight Loss

Herbal medicine is increasingly popular in the West, and is of great relevance to us. Herbs can be used to aid digestion, balance blood sugar levels and detox the body.

- Nettles and dandelion are diuretics that help to eliminate excess fluid.
- Dandelion root tea or coffee can be drunk freely to help balance blood sugar levels and support the ridding of toxins from the liver. (It also has a slight laxative effect.)
- Milk thistle capsules protect the liver and help digest fats. (The liver is often under stress when the body breaks down fat and releases stored toxins from fat cells.)
- Camomile is a calming herb that balances blood sugar levels; it can be made into a tea on its own or mixed with herbs like valerian and lime flowers to help alleviate anxiety and stress.
- Gymnema sylvestra can be dropped on the tongue (1–2 ml) per day to reduce sugar cravings and for appetite control.
- Malabar tamarind (also called garcinia cambogia) is a fruit available in capsule form that has been show in trials to substantially reduce appetite.
- Cleavers (also called goosegrass), which can be drunk as a tea, is a detoxifying herb that cleanses the lymph glands and can be mixed with fennel seeds for its digestive and diuretic effects.
- Bladderwrack or kelp is rich in iodine and will help to stimulate a sluggish thyroid.

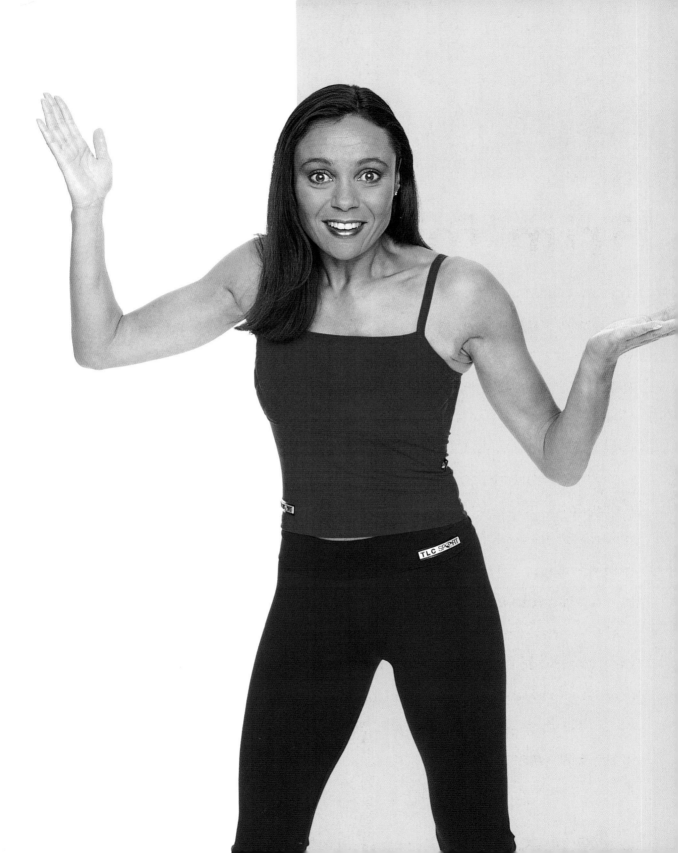

Chapter 6

Trim for Life

The final factor in the quest for a trim body is physical activity. If you are one of that increasing number of inactive individuals you need to consider changing your thinking about exercise. Many people think that being physically active means getting down to the gym and slogging it out on the treadmill. In fact there are many ways to enjoy using your body to get fit. Physical exercise brings numerous health benefits: it encourages the body to function better, boosts the metabolism, helps in the achievement and maintenance of your natural bodyweight, tones muscles and combats stress. It will also give you a natural high and promote a more positive state of mind. You can learn to love being physically active but first you need to make a conscious effort to be positive about it – to get started and then commit to doing it regularly and consistently. The more you do it the better you become at it. It's time to get moving and integrate physical activity into your daily life. So what do you need to do to achieve and maintain a trim body?

Trim for Life

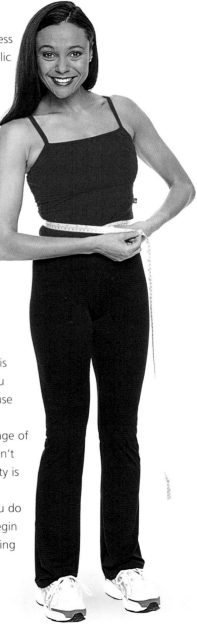

For a trim body shape you need to burn calories to get rid of the excess fat on your body. You can do this by exercising to boost your metabolic rate. Your metabolic rate (or the rate at which you burn energy) is affected by a number of different factors.

How active are you – completely inactive, moderately active or very active? How many of the above can you incorporate into your life? When will you start?

Body Composition

Your muscles are metabolically active even when you are resting; fat is considerably less so. The more muscle you have the more calories you will burn. Men generally have faster metabolisms than women because they have more muscle mass. Your age also affects your metabolism. Metabolic rate peaks at age 20 and declines thereafter. Around the age of 30 you start to lose muscle mass and your body fat increases. But don't blame old age for slowing you down or for making you fat – inactivity is the culprit. If you are inactive and you don't use your muscles they decrease in size and lose their shape as your metabolism slows. If you do the right amount of activity you can combat this process. You can begin to boost your metabolic rate by becoming more active and simply using your body as nature meant it to be used.

You can boost your metabolic rate by becoming more active.

Think about the following:

- Do you really need to travel everywhere by car? Walk as much as you can. If you do drive, park some way from where you are headed to give yourself a walk. If you drive to the supermarket, pick the spot in the car park farthest away from the entrance.
- Carry your shopping to the car instead of wheeling it in the trolley.
- Wear comfortable shoes so that you can move faster.
- Invest in a bicycle – you can use a backpack or a basket for shopping.
- Take the stairs instead of the lift. Begin by walking up the stairs and as you become fitter go faster or take two steps at a time – brilliant for your legs.
- Avoid using the remote control. Make the effort to haul yourself out of your chair and over to the TV to change channels.
- After eating, go for a walk around the block or just around the house to get your digestion working.
- Do the cleaning with gusto. As you vacuum make long, rhythmic movements. Make sure you lift chairs and get behind the sofa. Heavy housework burns 170 calories per hour.
- Get creative in your garden. Use a manual lawn mower. Don't buy an electric hedge trimmer – use shears and secateurs. Plant your own organic vegetable patch. Clear your leaves with a rake. Get on your hands and knees to do some weeding. Heavy gardening burns around 370 calories per hour.
- What else can you think of to boost your metabolism?

I have known many clients to lose their excess pounds by doing one or all of the above. Do likewise and you'll have made a great start. By putting into action a specific exercise programme you can further boost your metabolic rate and burn more calories so helping you reach your target weight faster.

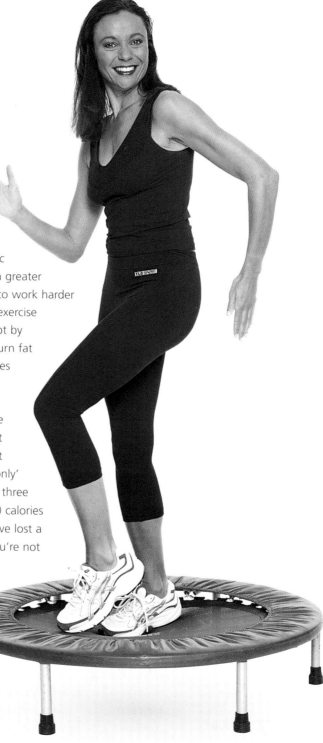

Aerobic Fitness

Aerobic fitness is a measure of your cardiovascular system's ability to deliver oxygen to the working muscles. Improving it involves using the major muscles of the body in large, rhythmic movements. This makes the body demand a greater volume of oxygen and the heart and lungs to work harder so they can meet that demand. And if you exercise regularly and consistently your muscles adapt by becoming more and more toned and you burn fat more effectively – in short, aerobic work gives your metabolism a boost.

Some people say that the effort an aerobic workout takes is not worth it for the few calories that you burn. It may seem that way, but it is how regularly you exercise that makes all the difference. Even if you burn 'only' 200 calories in a 30-minute aerobic session, three sessions a week is 600 calories. That is 2400 calories a month. Multiply by that by 12 and you have lost a good few pounds of fat over a year. And you're not just losing weight; exercise is well worth it for all the other benefits it brings: stronger heart and lungs, stronger muscles, better posture, stronger bones, improved psychological well-being, the relief of tension. The benefits of aerobic exercise should not be underestimated.

Write your own aerobic exercise programme for weight loss; set down how many times a week you'll work out, what you'll do and for how long. Make it realistic and achievable: a programme you will be able to follow consistently. Make a commitment to monitor the intensity of your workout.

The muscles use two systems for calorie burning. The aerobic system is where the fuel that is used is predominately fat broken down in the presence of oxygen. The aerobic system is capable of generating large amounts of energy because fat and oxygen are there in abundance. Together they work to burn calories, which is crucial for reducing body fat. The other system is the anaerobic system, which produces energy without oxygen. Its source of fuel is carbohydrates, which when broken down are stored in the muscles and liver as glycogen. The anaerobic system kicks in when the intensity of an activity increases to the point at which the aerobic system cannot supply enough oxygen to meet the body's energy demands.

Current thinking holds that low-intensity, long-duration activities are not necessarily the best for burning calories. High-intensity exercise burns calories as effectively and speeds the metabolism. But the intensity of a workout is, of course, relative to the individual. Walking at a brisk pace may represent high-intensity exercise for a beginner but a fitter person would need to go running to enjoy high-intensity exercise benefits. The longer or harder you work out, the more calories you burn and it is the total amount of calories lost that counts. As your fitness level increases, your body becomes even more efficient at burning calories and processing oxygen.

I would suggest that you work at an intensity that challenges but suits you. Complete beginners should focus on building up their workout to 20–30 minutes of aerobic activity four times a week to reduce body fat. Once you have reached your target, maintain those fitness levels by exercising aerobically two to three times a week. When you become fitter you can increase the intensity of your workout, change the type of workout, and increase the length of your workout. If you persevere you will experience the many benefits that exercise can bring you. Your body will learn to metabolize fat more efficiently, and you will achieve your target weight and simply feel great.

There are numerous activities to choose from if you want to get fit. The following list includes both aerobic and anaerobic activities. You simply have to choose the ones you will enjoy.

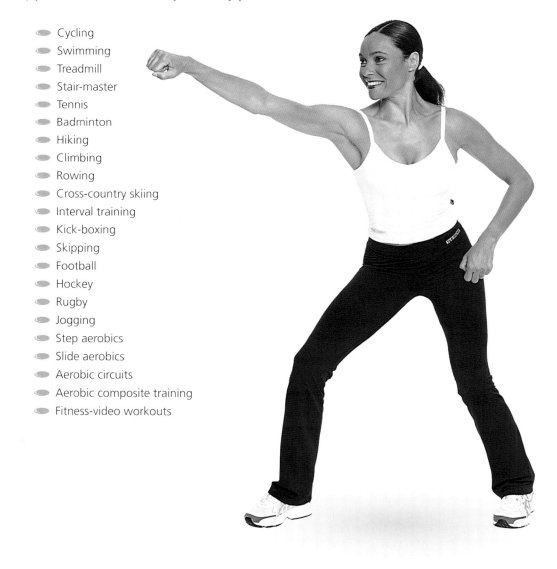

- Cycling
- Swimming
- Treadmill
- Stair-master
- Tennis
- Badminton
- Hiking
- Climbing
- Rowing
- Cross-country skiing
- Interval training
- Kick-boxing
- Skipping
- Football
- Hockey
- Rugby
- Jogging
- Step aerobics
- Slide aerobics
- Aerobic circuits
- Aerobic composite training
- Fitness-video workouts

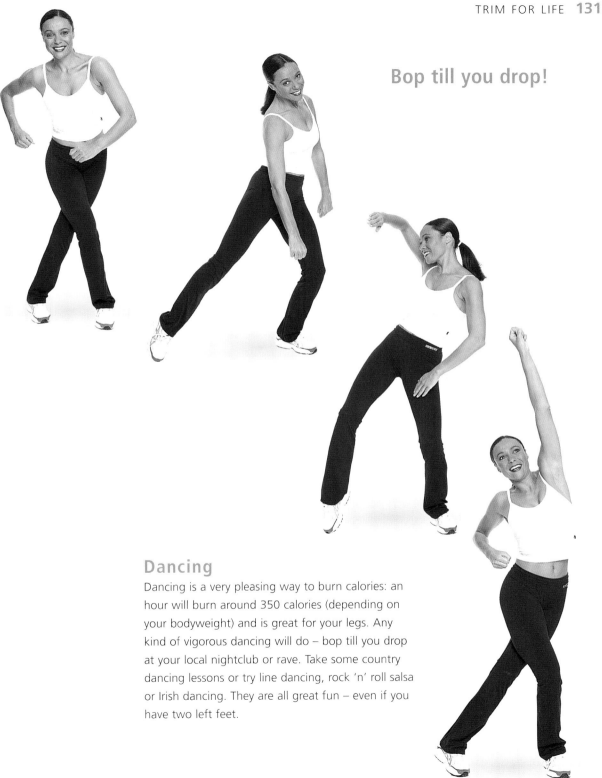

Bop till you drop!

Dancing

Dancing is a very pleasing way to burn calories: an hour will burn around 350 calories (depending on your bodyweight) and is great for your legs. Any kind of vigorous dancing will do – bop till you drop at your local nightclub or rave. Take some country dancing lessons or try line dancing, rock 'n' roll salsa or Irish dancing. They are all great fun – even if you have two left feet.

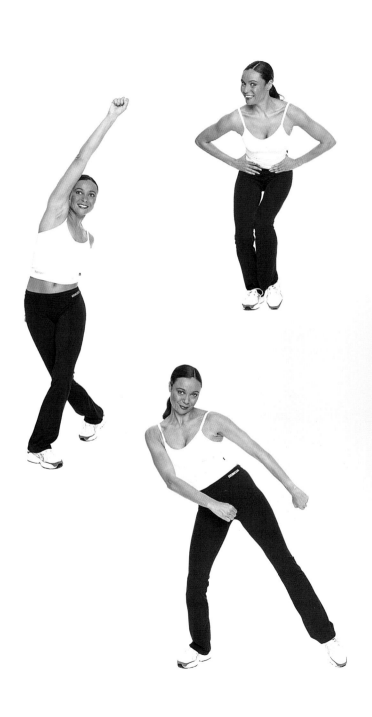

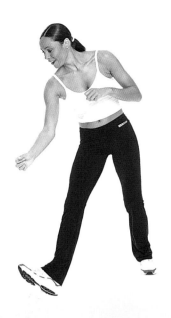

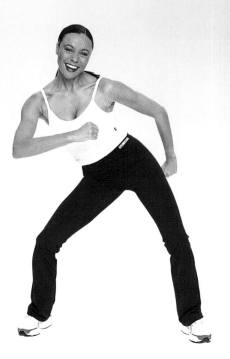

**Dancing is great fun –
even if you have two
left feet.**

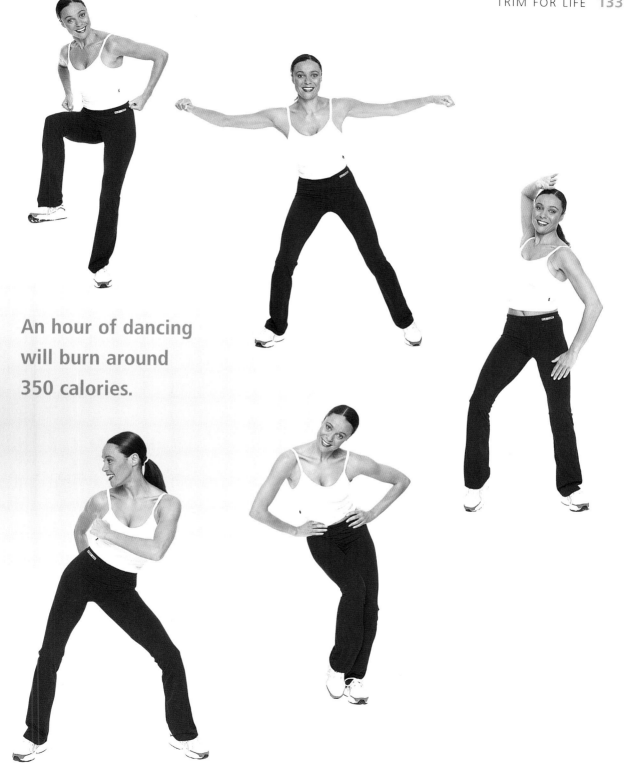

An hour of dancing
will burn around
350 calories.

Strength Work

Muscle is active tissue; it uses a large amount of energy even at rest. Inactivity causes muscles to decrease in strength as well as in size; and with a decrease in muscle mass the metabolic rate starts to slow down, which in turn leads to an increase in body fat. Strength exercise means working your muscles against resistance. By doing this you are increasing your metabolism by stimulating your muscles to become stronger and larger so that more calories are burned. Working against resistance will help you to maintain and build muscle throughout life, so that the musculoskeletal system stays balanced and tight. This promotes good posture and helps prevent injuries.

There are two different expressions of strength: the first defines strength as the maximum amount of force a muscle produces to overcome a resistance; the second, muscular endurance, reflects the muscles' ability to perform repeated actions over a period of time. Muscular endurance is increased alongside gains in muscular strength, so the two are related.

Strength training requires the exercising individual or specific groups of muscles against progressive resistance weight. When a muscle is worked against resistance it is stimulated into growing thereby increasing the size and strength of muscle fibres and resulting in a firm, sculpted look. Strength training

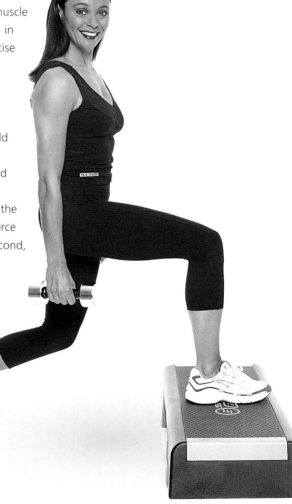

plays a major role in enhancing body shape. When you are trimming your body you have two choices: you can work on strength, which will give you a strong, sculpted body; or you can work on endurance, which will give you more tone.

When you exercise you work in repetitions (known as 'reps') and sets. Repetitions are the number of times you repeat a movement; sets are a group of repetitions. (So, if you're doing press-ups, two sets of 20 reps means 40 press-ups in total performed in two blocks of 20.) If you want to work for strength you do fewer repetitions against a higher resistance and vice versa for endurance. But note that there is no chance of bulking up for women because we don't have the same levels of testosterone in our bodies as men. Whichever way you work you will get a strong, toned body. The more resistance you apply to your muscles the more sculpted they become.

The complete beginner should start with minimum resistance to learn to exercise with good form and perfect technique. Each exercise should be performed slowly. At the beginning you need to focus on developing kinaesthetic awareness of how your exercise feels – it is while you are learning the technique you fix the habits of a lifetime. You also need to focus on breathing evenly and rhythmically throughout each rep, exhaling on the effort.

How can you increase your muscle mass and maintain it throughout your lifetime? Make a list of ways you can do this.

Research suggests that you get no further increase in strength by doing more than one set of an exercise. I am of the school of thought that believes two are better, developing greater muscle strength and tone and burning more calories.

You can increase your muscle mass through activities such as weight training (working with free weights or the machines and gadgets at the gym) or you can use your own bodyweight for resistance, or – somewhere between the two – you can use dynabands (rubber bands that increase the body's natural resistance; they are excellent if you're travelling). You can even use water as resistance.

Muscle Fatigue

As with aerobics, you must work at a pace that is challenging but safe. If you find yourself doing endless reps then you're not working hard enough; but equally if you work with too much resistance you could hurt yourself.

For a sculpted look, aim for 8 to 12 reps of an exercise; for a toned look work up to 15 reps. You will feel your muscles becoming overloaded – they feel tired and you feel like you can't do another rep – during the last reps of an exercise. You may get some muscle soreness following exercise. This is fairly common. If you are so sore and stiff that you can hardly move, clearly you have overdone it. Your muscles should feel pleasantly challenged and tired.

Stretching

This may not directly reduce the amount of fat on your body; however, it is an essential part of any exercise programme. You stretch to prepare the muscle for exercise; you stretch after exercise to prevent muscle tightness and shortening, which can decrease your range of movement. Focus on static stretching: these are stretches that you hold. Hold each one for a minimum of ten seconds and for longer if you wish to increase your flexibility. Make sure you stretch all the muscle groups that you have worked. Lastly, after all this thinking and doing to get yourself trim, stretch to relax.

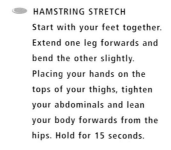

HAMSTRING STRETCH

Start with your feet together. Extend one leg forwards and bend the other slightly. Placing your hands on the tops of your thighs, tighten your abdominals and lean your body forwards from the hips. Hold for 15 seconds.

Stretching is an essential part of any exercise programme.

FRONT THIGH STRETCH

You may need a chair for support. Stand with your feet together. Shift your weight on to one leg and soften the knee. Bring the heel of the opposite leg up towards your buttocks and reach for the ankle. Tighten your abdominals and hold on to the ankle, tuck your pelvis under and make sure your knee faces the floor. Hold the stretch for 15 seconds.

CALF STRETCH

You may need a chair for support. Take a step forward with your right leg and bend the right knee. Make sure the left leg is straight with the heel pressed to the floor. Make sure the toes of both feet are facing forward and that a diagonal line runs from the heel of the back foot to the top of your head. Ensure your hips are facing forward. Hold the stretch for 15 seconds.

BUTTOCK STRETCH

Use a chair for support. Bend your supporting leg slightly. Bring the ankle of the opposite leg up and across the knee of the supporting leg, so that it looks as if you are crossing your legs standing up. Allow your upper body to lean forwards. Hold the stretch for 15 seconds.

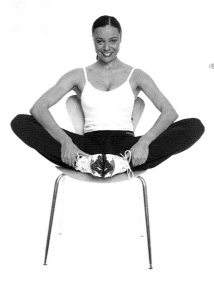

Stretch to relax.

INNER THIGH STRETCH

Sit on a chair with your back straight. Bend your knees and bring up the soles of your feet and press them together. Hold the stretch for 15 seconds.

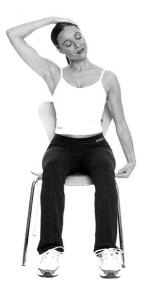

NECK STRETCH

In a sitting position drop your right ear towards your right shoulder. Bring your right arm over your right shoulder and press your head towards the right shoulder. Hold the stretch for 15 seconds.

Index

Bibliography

Bean, Anita, *The Complete Guide to Sports Nutrition,* A & C Black, 2000

Bovey, Shelley, *What Have You Got to Lose*, The Women's Press Ltd, 2002

Clarke, Jane, *Body Foods for Women,* Orion, 1997

Her Majesty's Stationery Office, *Tackling Obesity in England*, 2001–2002

Holford, Patrick, *Natural Highs,* Piatkus Books, 2001

Kenton, Leslie, *The X-factor Diet*, Vermilion, 2002

Krasner, Dr. A. M., *The Wizard Within*, American Board of Hypnotherapy, Press, 1990

McDermott, Ian and O'Connor, Joseph, *NLP and Health,* HarperCollins, 1996

Orbach, Sue, *Fat is a Feminest Issue,* Arrow, 1998

Reader's Digest, *Marvels and Mysteries of the Human Mind*, 1992

Sharon, Michael Dr., *Complete Nutrition,* Prion Books Ltd, 1997

Tebbetts, Charles, *Self Hypnosis and Other Mind Expanding Techniques*, Westwood Publishing, 1987

Other Resources

www.eda.uk.com (Eating Disorders Association)

www.fitnessworld.com

www.toast-uk.org (The Obesity and Awareness Trust)

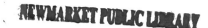

Acknowledgements

I would very much like to thank Carole Symons BSC (Hons) Medical Herbalist and Nutritional Advisor for being my nutritional consultant in this book. You can tap into her website www.herbalistuk.com. Thanks also to Simone Parkinson for her GI tables as well as the British Diabetic Association. Thanks also to NLP Master Practitioner Michael Kaufmann for his support. Thanks to Atkinson Ball College of Hypnotherapy for allowing me to adapt the appetite control exercise and to its training Seminar on NLP. To Ian Mcdermott for teaching me the foundations of NLP. Thanks to Jackie Strachen and Mark Smith who have given me the opportunity to write this book and to Victoria Alers-Hankey for her enthusiasm. Thanks to my agent Vicki McIvor for her help.

Thanks also to Bill Morton and his photographic team for the pictures in this book also to Martyn Fletcher for the wonderful make up. Thanks to The fitness Network for their fitness apparatus. As ever I am extremely grateful to the Leotard Company for providing the stunning outfits. You can receive a mail order catalogue from The Thatch, Great Billing Park, Northampton NN3. Many thanks to Pissarro's on the River for allowing us to photograph in their lovely restaurant. Lastly, as always, many thanks to my friends and family for their support throughout the writing of this book.